DIABETIC GOODIE BOOK

by Kathy Kochan

First Edition

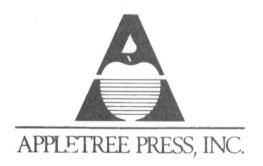

APPLETREE PRESS, INC.

Mankato, MN

Appletree Press Inc.
151 Good Counsel Drive Suite 125
Mankato, MN 56001
Phone #507-345-4848
Fax #507-345-3002

The reader is cautioned to consult with his or her physician and/or registered dietitian prior to consuming or serving any of the foods produced in this cookbook. Keep in mind that just because these recipes are lower in calories, it doesn't mean the reader can double the servings he/she eats. The recipes given in this text were developed to help readers/cooks adopt a heart-healthy, carbohydrate-controlled eating pattern and are not intended as a substitute for any treatment prescribed by a physician. This book is intended as a reference and cooking book only, not as a medical guide for self-treatment.

Acknowledgment: Recipes copyright© 1992 by Kathy Kochan as "De-Lite-Ful Desserts."
First Edition, first printing: 5,000 copies

Cataloging-in-Publication Data
Kochan, Kathy, 1949-.
Diabetic goodie book : don't cheat your sweet tooth / Kathy Kochan ; editors, Linda Hachfeld and Faith Winchester. Mankato, MN : Appletree Press, c1996.

256 p. ; 30 cm.
Includes glossary and index

Summary: Over 150 dessert and baked goods recipes each controlled for carbohydrate, fat, cholesterol and sodium. Recipes are appropriate for persons following a diabetic, heart-healthy or weight-control program. Nutrient profile, food exchanges and carbohydrate counting included.

ISBN 0-9620471-7-1

1. Diabetes—Diet therapy—Recipes. 2. Desserts. 3. Low-fat diet—Recipes. I. Title. II. Don't cheat your sweet tooth.

RC662   96-086653
641.5/6314   CIP

Nutrition Editor: Linda Hachfeld
Design & Layout Editor: Faith Winchester
Cover Design/Artwork: Kath Christensen Graphic Design

Prin   States

Dedication

I wish to dedicate this, my first cookbook, to the men in my life:
My husband Hank and my sons David and Marc.
Without their love, support, patience and willingness
to try anything once, this book would never have been created.

Table of Contents

Foreword

What a delight to work with such varied recipes as are found in the DIABETIC GOODIE BOOK. For some time now, I have wanted to see a recipe book with typically-enjoyed desserts such as cookies, cakes and crisps that are sensitive to the total amount of carbohydrate and fat. Goodies that are controlled in both nutrients can be enjoyed by anyone concerned about managing their weight or maintaining good cardiovascular health, as well as by healthy individuals with diabetes.

In 1994, nutritional recommendations changed drastically. Scientific evidence showed that sucrose (table sugar) as part of a mealplan could be used by individuals with type I or type II diabetes, without sacrificing blood glucose control. In other words, a carbohydrate is a carbohydrate whether it comes from a glass of milk, a cookie or a serving of potatoes. It is much more important to know the total amount of carbohydrate than its source. For more information on carbohydrates, carbohydrate counting and the exchange lists please refer to pages 229-230.

What makes Kathy Kochan's recipes so special is that she has worked diligently for years to develop tasty recipes using small amounts of sugar (usually no more than 1/4 cup per recipe), whole grains and nonfat or low-fat ingredients. Oftentimes, she reduces preparation time by using the food processor and the microwave.

All of her cheesecakes and scones and most of her cookies, quick breads, fruit desserts and pies can easily be counted as 1 or 2 carbohydrate choices. Here are some delicious examples of recipes that count as one carbohydrate choice: Layered Cheesecake Squares, Peach Snowcaps, Easy & Flaky Apple Turnovers, Crustless Pumpkin Pie, Island Muffins, Blueberry Cornmeal Scones, Delightful Butter Cookies or Chocolate Cloud Cake.

May you enjoy making these great tasting recipes for yourself and others. I think you'll agree with me that they are worth the effort, and you'll receive rave reviews.

Linda Hachfeld, MPH, RD
Author of COOKING ALA HEART

Introduction

One of my favorite pastimes is cooking and baking. Having diabetes since the age of 5, eating everything I want is impossible. I look forward to dessert after dinner and refuse to watch everyone else enjoy their desserts while I munch on a piece of plain fruit.

Since I enjoy spending time in the kitchen, I developed recipes that I can eat without feeling guilty and can serve my family and guests. The recipes in DIABETIC GOODIE BOOK call for low-fat ingredients, small amounts of sugar and little or no added salt. This cookbook is designed for people who are interested in having desserts and baked goods while maintaining a healthy eating plan.

Each person needs to take responsibility for his and her own health. Whether or not you have diabetes, food must be tasty, nourishing and easy to prepare. Healthy people with diabetes can incorporate sugar into recipes as long as carbohydrates are calculated and worked into their meal plan. Most of the recipes in this book are prepared with fruit for natural sugar and sweetness, since I personally do not use artificial sweeteners. The majority of the desserts and baked goods in this cookbook call for small amounts of sugar and fat. The recipes are also easy and fast to prepare when using the microwave.

My family enjoys entertaining, and the recipes in DIABETIC GOODIE BOOK are terrific for guests. Many of our friends and acquaintances are concerned about what they eat. By incorporating fiber into the recipes through the use of whole-wheat flour and fresh fruit, you'll find these desserts and baked goods more filling and satisfying. Fruits are rich in fiber, contribute a variety of vitamins and minerals to our daily diet and yet are low in calories.

While I taught cooking classes, I learned from my students what people really wanted in a cookbook: simple instructions on how to prepare healthy, tasty food quickly and easily. I have done my best in writing this cookbook with recipes which fulfill this requirement.

So, grab an apron, wash your hands and get started. Surprise your family, your guests and yourself with a delectable dessert that's good for everyone. I'm sure you will agree these are the most delightful goodies you have ever enjoyed!

Kathy Kochan, Author

Handy Tips From Kathy's Kitchen

Foods

When beating egg whites: separate eggs right from the refrigerator. Let stand at room temperature at least a half hour before attempting to beat. Be sure beaters and bowl do not contain a bit of fat which will inhibit the whites from foaming and beating stiff. Do not use a plastic bowl. Plastics are impossible to rid of fat.

Use a small funnel to separate cold eggs. Open the egg over the funnel and the white will run through and the yolk will remain. Brown and white eggs are the same quality.

If you shake an egg and hear a rattle, it's stale. A fresh egg will float and a stale one will sink.

Dried lemon and orange peels may be purchased in the spice section of the food store. Read label to be sure to purchase unsweetened.

Pie crust pastry is the most caloric part of any pie. Chill at least 1 hour before rolling so it can be rolled extra thin. Discard the excess dough.

Do not wash any type of berries until just before using. Hull strawberries after they are washed and drained.

When using fresh fruit in a recipe, use only ripe fruits. They will be more flavorful because of the natural sugar. The riper they are, the sweeter they usually taste. To ripen fruit: place in paper bag, close loosely and store at room temperature. It is ripe when fruit gives gently to pressure and smells sweet. Refrigerate until needed.

Try not to peel fruit. Washed fruit skins are high in natural fiber. If you prefer to peel: plunge peaches into boiling water for 20 seconds, drain and run under cold water. Peel should slide off.

Extra ripe bananas can be peeled and frozen in plastic bags. Defrost and use in baking.

If baked goods are not rising, check the freshness of your baking powder. Mix 1 teaspoon with 1/3 cup hot water. If mixture does not foam, the powder is stale and should not be used. Purchase a new container.

If brown sugar is rock hard, add a slice of soft bread to the package, close tightly, and in a few hours the sugar will be soft again. Remove bread and store tightly covered.

To soften butter or margarine, unwrap and place on a plate and microwave on high for 15 to 20 seconds.

To drain yogurt: place yogurt in 2 coffee filters over a sturdy measuring cup or small bowl and refrigerate covered; allow to drain 2 to 24 hours or until yogurt is the desired consistency. Discard whey (liquid which has drained). Store yogurt cheese covered in refrigerator. Whey may continue releasing, just pour off any accumulated liquid before using.

When you have the time, chop walnuts and pecans and store in a plastic bag or a container in the refrigerator. When a recipe calls for chopped nuts, they will be available.

Keep shelled and chopped nuts in refrigerator. They will keep indefinitely. Nuts can also be frozen.

To lower the amount of fat in baked goods containing nuts, decrease the amount of chopped nuts used by toasting them. Toasted nuts have more flavor and therefore you can use less. To toast nuts: place chopped nuts on baking sheet and bake 3 to 5 minutes in a preheated 350°F. Cool before stirring into batter. You can also toast nuts and store in a covered container or plastic bag until ready to use.

Tools
Spray measuring cup with cooking spray before measuring molasses or honey.

Snip dates with a scissors used specifically for food. Wet scissors or spray with cooking spray before snipping dates.

Use an ice cream scoop to fill cupcake papers without spilling.

Safety & Cleanliness
Always wash hands well before working with food. Be sure counter and cooking and baking utensils are clean and in good condition.

Use a damp paper towel to wipe off all cans before opening the tops. Also wipe blades on can opener after each use.

Wash unpeeled fruit before eating or using in a recipe.

Use sharp knives to prevent injuries.

Wrap foods airtight and label before placing in freezer. Remove all air when wrapping. Use oldest items first. See page 238 for freezer storage times.

Store opened containers of yogurt, cottage cheese, cream cheese or ricotta cheese upside down on a saucer. The cheese product will stay fresher longer. Discard any liquid that drains into saucer.

Trim, peel and scrape foods over waxed paper for easy cleanup.

Keep a damp cloth close at hand for a quick cleanup. Wipe off counter, range and microwave each time you use it.

Wash utensils as you work. There will be less cleanup afterwards.

Measuring Ingredients
Cans of skim milk and egg substitute: shake before measuring.

All-purpose and whole wheat flours: stir to aerate flour and spoon into the measuring cup then level off with spatula.

Baking powder, baking soda, cream of tartar and spices: dip and fill measuring spoon then level off with spatula.

Brown sugar: spoon into measuring cup and pack down firmly then level off with spatula.

Sugar: spoon into measuring cup then level off with spatula.

Cake flour: spoon lightly into measuring cup then level off with spatula.

Egg: use large eggs

Liquids: pour into a measuring cup designed for liquids, place on counter and check measurements at eye level.

When sifting whole wheat flour, grains will remain in sifter. Simply add to flour already sifted.

Measures

Dash	Liquid: few drops Dry: less than 1/8 tsp
3 tsp	1 Tbs
1 1/2 tsp	1/2 Tbs
4 Tbs	1/4 cup
5 Tbs plus 1 tsp	1/3 cup
8 Tbs	1/2 cup
10 Tbs plus 2 tsp	2/3 cup
12 Tbs	3/4 cup
16 Tbs	1 cup
2 cups	1 pint
4 cups (2 pints)	1 quart
4 quarts liquid	1 gallon
1 fluid ounce	2 Tbs
8 fluid ounces	1 cup
32 fluid ounces	1 quart

Approximate Yields

1 lb light butter or light margarine	2 cups
1 lb nonfat cottage cheese	2 cups
15 ounces nonfat ricotta cheese	2 cups
4 large eggs	1 cup
8 to 10 large egg whites	1 cup
14 to 16 large egg yolks	1 cup
10 4-inch graham crackers	1 cup crumbs
1 lemon	2 tsp grated rind or dried peel or 2-3 Tbs juice
1 orange	2 Tbs grated rind or dried peel or 1/3 cup juice
1 lb raisins or snipped dates	3 cups
1 lb shelled almonds or pecans	4 cups
1 lb walnuts	3 cups
1 lb apples (3 medium)	3 cups sliced
1 lb bananas (3-4 medium)	2 cups mashed
1 pint blueberries	2 cups
1 lb peaches/nectarines (4 medium)	3 cups sliced
1 lb plums (4 medium)	3 cups sliced
1 pint strawberries	4 cups whole, 2 cups sliced or pureed
1 lb carrots	3-3 1/2 cups shredded

Utensils Needed for Recipes

Measuring cups for dry ingredients: 1/4, 1/3, 1/2 and 1 cup

Measuring cup for liquid ingredients

4-cup glass measuring cup

Measuring spoons/teaspoons

Rubber and metal spatulas

Wooden spoons

Whisks: small, medium and large

Bowls: small, large and very large

Food processor or blender

Electric mixer

Can opener

Cutting board

Paring knife

Vegetable peeler

Serrated knife

Strainer

9-inch tart pan with removable rim

13 x 9 x 2-inch pan

10-inch tube or bundt pan

8- or 9-inch spring form pan

15 x 10 x1-inch jelly roll pan

8- and 9-inch square pans

8- and 9-inch round pans

10-inch pie plate

Metal muffin baking tins

Miniature muffin baking tins

Loaf pans: 3x5, 3x7, 5x8, 5x9

Baking or cookie sheets

2-quart casserole dish

Wire rack

Pot holders

Substitutions
for Recipes in this Book

Olive Oil or Canola Oil — These oils are used in the recipes and are good sources of monounsaturated fats. Your favorite vegetable oil could also be substituted; safflower, sunflower, corn and soybean oils are polyunsaturated fats. All are liquid at room temperature.

Buttermilk — Dry buttermilk powder can be substituted. Use 1 tablespoon of dry buttermilk powder and 1/4 cup water for each 1/4 cup of liquid buttermilk required in a recipe. Dry buttermilk powder should be mixed with dry ingredients and the required amount of water should be mixed with wet ingredients. Store opened containers of dry buttermilk powder in refrigerator. One brand, *Saco Dry Buttermilk*, can be purchased in most food stores and is located in the same aisle as flour and sugar.

If buttermilk is not available, use sour milk. To make sour milk, put lemon juice or white vinegar in a glass measuring cup. (See measurements below.) Add enough skim milk to equal the amount of sour milk required; stir. Wait about 3 minutes for milk to curdle; stir. Proceed as directed in the recipe.

To make:	Use:
1 cup or 3/4 cup sour milk	1 Tbs lemon juice or white vinegar
1/2 cup sour milk	2 tsp lemon juice or white vinegar
1/3 cup sour milk	1 1/2 tsp lemon juice or white vinegar

Egg Substitute — There are several brand names that can be found in the freezer or refrigerator sections of food stores. If you choose to use whole eggs or eggs whites, use this substitution guideline:
1/4 cup egg substitute = 1 whole egg = 2 egg whites.

Pasteurized Dried Egg White — This is necessary when the recipe requiring eggs/egg whites is not cooked or baked, as in many puddings, unbaked cheesecakes and meringue recipes. If using the product *Just Whites*, use these substitution guidelines: For 1 egg white, use 2 tsp of Just Whites and 2 Tbs WARM water. If using Instant Meringue Mix, 1 packet is the equivalent of 3 egg whites and should be mixed with 1/3 cup COLD water.

Check label directions before using any product.

How To Tackle A Recipe

❑ Read the recipe all the way through before starting.

❑ Check your supplies to see if you have all the ingredients.

❑ Check to see that you have the right equipment; i.e. pans, electric mixer, etc.

❑ Set out all ingredients and equipment. Follow directions exactly.

❑ Check the number of servings to meet your needs.

❑ Do as much preparation prior to combining ingredients; i.e. chopping, peeling, getting eggs to room temperature.

❑ Spray baking utensils with cooking spray instead of greasing and flouring them. Clean-up is also easier.

❑ Preheat oven for baking unless recipe tells you not to.

❑ Do not cut or increase recipes unless you are skilled enough to recognize the difference in pan sizes and/or cooking time necessitated by the change.

❑ When using a glass ovenproof baking dish, decrease oven temperature by 25° because the cake will brown faster.

Nutrition Information in the Recipes

DIABETIC GOODIE BOOK recipes were designed to help control amounts of carbohydrate, fat, cholesterol and sodium. Each nutrient analysis includes total calories, total carbohydrates, protein, total fat, cholesterol, sodium and fiber. The rounding rules established by the Food & Drug Administration have been used to the best of our ability in reporting the nutritional composition of the recipes. Food Exchanges as developed by the American Dietetic Association and the American Diabetes Association are also listed with each recipe. If an ingredient is listed as (optional) in the recipe, its nutrient value is NOT calculated in the nutrient profile or Exchanges. Please see pages 229-230 for more information on carbohydrate counting and Food Exchange Lists.

Cookies & Bars

For evenly browned cookies, use shiny, bright baking sheets at least 2 inches narrower and shorter than the oven. Spray pan with cooking spray only if recipe directs you to do so.

Always place dough on a cool baking sheet; dough spreads on a hot one. Try working with 3 or 4 baking sheets so you can fill and bake at the same time.

To mold cookies, roll dough between palms of hands. Be sure texture is smooth so cookies brown and have the correct texture.

Cookies should be removed from cookie sheet with a metal spatula and placed on racks to cool completely, about 10 minutes, before storing in a tightly covered container.

Discard old darkened baking sheets if cookies do not bake correctly. Purchase new ones to bake delicious, evenly-browned cookies.

If cookies do not seem to bake well, check oven temperature to be sure you are baking cookies at the correct temperature as stated in the recipe. If the oven is too hot or too cool, your cookies will not bake evenly. Use an oven thermometer to determine if your oven is gauged correctly.

When you want fresh, baked cookies in a flash, whip up a recipe for bar or square cookies. Such cookies take less time to make since you just mix and pat them into a pan. Many bars and squares require only one bowl for mixing and are baked in about 30 minutes. After about 10 minutes you can cut them into squares or 1x2-inch bars and serve. Most bars or squares are moist and should be stored tightly covered. Since they are cut, they do not retain their freshness as long as most cookies.

Some quick-fix bars include APPLE RAISIN BARS, CHOCOLATE JAM SQUARES, SIMPLE BANANA BARS, BANANAS POPPY SEED BARS, CHEWY COCONUT SQUARES, DEVILISHLY DELICIOUS CHOCOLATE BARS, MIX-IN-THE-PAN DATE BARS, DATE CHEWS and RASPBERRY BARS.

Refer to page 235 for reasons for imperfect cookies and pages 237-238 for hints and storage tips for freezing cookies and bars.

DELIGHTFUL BUTTER COOKIES

USE COLORED SUGAR FOR HOLIDAY BAKING
Prep time: 15 min   Bake time: 8-10 min
Makes: 48   Serving size: 3 Cookies
Exchanges: 1 Starch (1 Carbohydrate Choice)
Analysis per serving: 93 Calories, 15 g Carbohydrate, 2 g Protein,
2 g Fat, 7 mg Cholesterol, 84 mg Sodium, 1 g Fiber

1/2	cup (1 stick) light butter, softened
1/4	cup sugar
2	large egg whites or 1/4 cup egg substitute
1	cup all-purpose flour
1	cup whole-wheat flour
2	tsp baking powder
1	tsp dried orange peel or grated fresh orange peel
2	Tbs orange juice
1	tsp vanilla extract
	Plain or colored sugar

Preheat oven to 350°F. Spray baking sheets with cooking spray.

In a medium bowl, use electric mixer at medium speed to cream light butter; scrape sides.   Add sugar and beat until light and fluffy, scraping bowl occasionally. Add egg whites; beat well.

On waxed paper or in a small bowl, stir together flours, baking powder and orange peel. Beat in combined dry ingredients, juice and vanilla, scraping sides of bowl occasionally, until dough is thoroughly blended.

Using a teaspoon of dough per cookie, shape into balls and place 2 inches apart on prepared baking sheets. Spray bottom of a flat 2-inch glass with cooking spray and dip in sugar; flatten each cookie. Respray glass as necessary and dip in sugar for each cookie.

Bake 8 to 10 minutes or until browned around edges. Use a metal spatula to transfer cookies to racks to cool completely. When cool, store covered.

SCRUMPTIOUS PEANUT BUTTER COOKIES

THE PEANUT BUTTER LOVER'S COOKIE
Prep time: 20 min   Baking time: 10 min
Makes: 72   Serving size: 2 Cookies
Exchanges: 1/2 Starch and 1 Fat (1 Carbohydrate Choice)
Analysis per serving: 90 Calories, 10 g Carbohydrate, 3 g Protein,
5 g Fat, 3 mg Cholesterol, 62 mg Sodium, 1 g Fiber

1	cup all-purpose flour
1	cup whole-wheat flour
1	tsp baking soda
1	tsp baking powder
1/2	cup light butter or light margarine, softened
1	cup natural peanut butter
1/4	cup sugar
1/4	cup brown sugar
1	Tbs vanilla extract
4	large egg whites or 1/2 cup egg substitute
3	Tbs skim milk

Preheat oven to 375°F. Set out ungreased baking sheets.

Sift flours, baking soda and baking powder onto waxed paper or into small bowl. If grains remain in sifter, simply add to dry ingredients.

In large bowl, with electric mixer at medium speed, beat light butter, peanut butter and sugars until smooth; scrape sides. Beat in vanilla, egg whites and milk at medium speed until blended. Gradually add dry ingredients and beat at medium speed until well blended.

Using a teaspoonful of dough, shape into 1-inch balls and place 2-inches apart on baking sheet. Flatten with tines of fork, making crisscross design.

Bake 10 to 12 minutes or until lightly browned. Use a metal spatula to transfer cookies to wire rack to cool completely before storing in tightly covered container.

"MY WAY" CHOCOLATE CHIP COOKIES

ALMOST EVERYONE'S FAVORITE COOKIE
Prep time: 15 min   Bake time: 8 min
Makes: 48   Serving size: 2 Cookies
Exchanges: 1 Starch (1 Carbohydrate Choice)
Analysis per serving: 82 Calories, 13 g Carbohydrate, 1 g Protein,
3 g Fat, 14 mg Cholesterol, 45 mg Sodium, 1 g Fiber

1/2	cup (1 stick) light margarine or light butter, softened
2	Tbs sugar
1/4	cup brown sugar
1	large egg or 1/4 cup egg substitute
1/2	tsp vanilla extract
1	Tbs skim milk
1/2	cup old-fashioned oats
3/4	cup all-purpose flour
3/4	cup whole-wheat flour
1/2	tsp baking soda
1/2	cup mini chocolate chips

Heat oven to 375°F. Spray baking sheets with cooking spray.

In a large bowl, with electric mixer at medium speed, cream light margarine and sugars until light and fluffy; scrape sides of bowl. Beat in egg, vanilla and milk at medium speed; scrape sides.

In small bowl, combine oatmeal, flours and baking soda. Use a rubber spatula to stir into batter until well blended; stir in chips.

Drop by teaspoonfuls onto prepared baking sheets, spacing about 2 inches apart. Spray bottom of a flat 2-inch glass with cooking spray and use to flatten each cookie, respraying glass when necessary.

Bake 8 to 10 minutes or until lightly browned. Use a metal spatula to transfer cookies to a wire rack to cool completely. When cool, store tightly covered.

❖ To make bar cookies, add 1 tablespoon of orange juice to the batter and spread into a 13x9-inch pan which has been sprayed with cooking spray. Bake about 12 minutes or until browned. Cool about 10 minutes before cutting into 32 bars.

OUTRAGEOUS OATMEAL COOKIES

OUTRAGEOUSLY DELICIOUS
Prep time: 10 min   Bake time: 8 min
Makes: 72   Serving size: 3 Cookies
Exchanges: 1 Starch (1 Carbohydrate Choice)
Analysis per serving: 100 Calories, 15 g Carbohydrate, 3 g Protein,
3 g Fat, 5 mg Cholesterol, 102 mg Sodium, 2 g Fiber

1/3	**cup chopped nuts**
1	**cup whole-wheat flour**
1/4	**cup wheat germ**
1/4	**cup unprocessed bran**
1	**tsp cinnamon**
1/4	**tsp nutmeg**
1/8	**tsp ground cloves**
1/3	**cup nonfat dry milk powder**
1	**tsp baking soda**
1	**tsp baking powder**
1/2	**cup light margarine or light butter, softened**
1/2	**cup unsweetened applesauce**
1/2	**cup brown sugar**
4	**large egg whites or 1/2 cup egg substitute**
2	**cups old-fashioned oats**
1/4	**cup raisins**

Preheat oven to 350°F. Spray baking sheets with cooking spray.   Place nuts on baking sheet and bake 3 to 5 minutes or until toasted; set aside.

In medium bowl, use a rubber spatula to combine flour, wheat germ, bran, cinnamon, nutmeg, cloves, dry milk and baking powder; set aside.

In large bowl, with electric mixer at medium speed, beat light margarine, applesauce and sugar until light and fluffy. Add egg whites and beat at medium speed until well mixed, scraping sides of bowl. Gradually beat in flour mixture at low speed until blended, scraping bowl after each addition. Stir in oatmeal, toasted nuts and raisins until well blended.

Drop by rounded teaspoonfuls about 2 inches apart on prepared cookie sheets. If desired, spray bottom of a flat 2-inch glass with cooking spray and use to flatten each cookie. Bake 8 to 10 minutes or until lightly browned. Use a metal spatula to transfer cookies to a wire rack to cool completely. Store tightly covered.

SPECIAL SPICE COOKIES

CRISP SPICY COOKIES DELICIOUS DUNKED IN MILK
Prep time: 15 min   Bake time: 7 min
Makes: 48   Serving size: 2 Cookies
Exchanges: 1 Fruit and 1 Fat (1 Carbohydrate Choice)
Analysis per serving: 90 Calories, 11 g Carbohydrate, 1 g Protein,
5 g Fat, 8 mg Cholesterol, 97 mg Sodium, 1 g Fiber

1/2	cup olive or canola oil
1/4	cup molasses
2	Tbs sugar
1	large egg or 1/4 cup egg substitute
1	tsp butter extract (optional)
1	cup all-purpose flour
1	cup whole-wheat flour
2	tsp baking soda
1	tsp cinnamon
1/2	tsp ginger
1/2	tsp cloves

Preheat oven to 375°F. Spray baking sheets with cooking spray.

In a large bowl, using electric mixer at medium speed, beat oil, molasses, sugar, egg and butter extract, if using, until well blended.

In separate bowl, use a rubber spatula to combine flours, baking soda, cinnamon, ginger and cloves . With electric mixer at medium speed, gradually beat dry ingredients into molasses mixture until well blended, scraping bowl after each addition.

Form into 1-inch balls and place on prepared cookie sheet. Spray bottom of a 2-inch glass with cooking spray and dip in sugar and press each cookie ball with bottom of a glass. Respray and dip glass in sugar as needed until all balls are flattened.

Bake 7 to 10 minutes or until browned. Use a metal spatula to transfer cookies to a wire rack to cool completely. Store in a covered container.

FRUITY NUT COOKIES

A GREAT CHRISTMAS COOKIE SWEETENED ONLY BY FRUIT
Prep time: 90 min   Bake time: 15 min
Makes: 48   Serving size: 3 Cookies
Exchanges: 1 Fruit and 1 Fat (1 Carbohydrate Choice)
Analysis per serving: 100 Calories, 14 g Carbohydrate, 2 g Protein,
5 g Fat, 21 mg Cholesterol, 106 mg Sodium, 1 g Fiber

1/2	cup whole-wheat flour
1/2	cup all-purpose flour
1	tsp baking powder
1/4	tsp salt
1/2	cup light butter or light margarine, softened
2	tsp brandy or bourbon
1	large egg or 1/4 cup egg substitute
1	cup shredded coconut
1/4	cup raisins
1/2	cup chopped dates
1	cup chopped nuts (optional)

In large bowl, use a wooden spoon to mix flours, baking powder and salt.
Cut in butter with pastry blender or two knives scissor-fashion until
particles are pea-sized. Stir in remaining ingredients and mix with wooden
spoon or by hand until dough forms. Cover and chill 1 hour.

Preheat oven 350°F. Spray baking sheets with cooking spray. Shape
dough into 1-inch balls. With tines of fork dipped in flour, flatten balls with
a crisscross pattern.

Bake about 15 minutes or until lightly brown. Use a metal spatula to
transfer cookies to a wire rack to cool completely. Store tightly covered.

❖ If desired, toast nuts at 350°F for about 5 minutes or until browned.
Cool nuts before adding to batter. Toasted nuts are more flavorful.

SPICY NUT CLOUDS

FUNNY-LOOKING COOKIES THAT ARE LIGHT AS AIR
Prep time: 15 min   Bake time: 35 min
Makes: 36   Serving size: 2 Cookies
Exchanges: 1/2 Fruit and 1 Fat (1 Carbohydrate Choice)
Analysis per serving: 66 Calories, 7 g Carbohydrate, 1 g Protein,
4 g Fat, 0 mg Cholesterol, 7 mg Sodium, 0 g Fiber

1	cup finely chopped walnuts
1/2	cup sugar
1	tsp cinnamon
1/4	tsp nutmeg
1/4	tsp ground cloves
2	large egg whites, at room temperature

Preheat oven to 350°F. Place nuts on baking sheet and bake 3 to 5 minutes or until toasted. Set aside until cool.

Lower oven to 275°F. Line baking sheets with aluminum foil or parchment paper.

In small bowl, combine sugar and spices; set aside.

In large bowl, use electric mixer to beat egg whites at high speed until frothy. Gradually beat in spicy sugar mixture at high speed, scraping bowl after each addition until stiff peaks form when batter is lifted with a rubber spatula. Use spatula to gently fold in nuts.

Drop by teaspoonfuls onto prepared baking sheets. Bake 20 to 25 minutes until golden brown and crisp. Immediately transfer aluminum foil or parchment paper with cookies to wire rack to cool for 5 minutes, then remove cookies from foil and cool completely. Store in a tightly covered container.

❖ Do not make on a humid or rainy day because they will not be light in texture.

CHOCOLATE CLOUDS

THEY MELT IN YOUR MOUTH
Prep time: 15 min   Bake time: 30 min
Makes: 36   Serving size: 3 Cookies
Exchanges: 1/2 Fruit (1 Carbohydrate Choice)
Analysis per serving: 36 Calories, 9 g Carbohydrte, 1 g Protein,
0 g Fat, 0 mg Cholesterol, 58 mg Sodium, 0 g Fiber

2	large egg whites, at room temperature
1/2	cup sugar
1/4	tsp salt
1/4	tsp cream of tartar
1	tsp vanilla extract
1	Tbs cocoa

Preheat oven to 275°F. Line 2 baking sheets with aluminum foil or parchment paper.

In medium bowl, with electric mixer at high speed, beat egg whites until frothy. Beat in salt and cream of tartar at high speed until soft peaks form when batter is lifted with rubber spatula. Gradually add sugar and continue beating at high speed until peaks are stiff.   Scrape sides of bowl and beat in vanilla at high speed. Use rubber spatula to gently fold in cocoa until well blended.

Drop by teaspoonfuls onto prepared cookie sheets. Bake 30 to 35 minutes. Immediately remove aluminum foil or parchment paper with baked cookies to rack. Cool 1 minute and remove cookies from foil and cool completely on rack. Store in covered container.

❖ Do not make on a humid or rainy day because they will not be light. If desired, stir 1/4 cup semi-sweet mini chocolate chips or 1/2 cup chopped reduced-fat chocolate chips into batter along with cocoa. Proceed as directed.

ANISE BISCOTTI

A FLAVORFUL COOKIE PERFECT FOR DUNKING
Prep time: 30 min   Bake time: 35 min
Makes: 40   Serving size: 2 Biscotti
Exchanges: 1 Starch (1 Carbohydrate Choice)
Analysis per serving: 85 Calories, 14 g Carbohydrate, 2 g Protein,
2 g Fat, 10 mg Cholesterol, 51 mg Sodium, 0 g Fiber

1/2	cup sugar
3	Tbs olive or canola oil
1	large egg
1	large egg white
1 1/2	tsp dried orange peel or grated fresh orange peel
1	tsp vanilla extract
2	cups all-purpose flour,divided
3/4	tsp baking powder
1/4	tsp salt
2	tsp anise seeds

Preheat oven to 325°F. Spray a baking sheet with cooking spray.

In large bowl, with electric mixer at medium speed, combine sugar, oil, egg, egg white, orange peel and vanilla until well blended, scraping sides of bowl occasionally.

In a small bowl, combine 1 3/4 cup of flour with baking powder, salt and anise seeds and add to mixture. Beat at medium speed until well blended. Beat in enough of remaining flour to make a soft dough.

Turn dough out onto a lightly floured surface; divide dough in half. Shape into two 12-inch rolls; place on cookie sheets and flatten rolls to 1/2-inch thickness.

Bake for 25 minutes. Lower oven to 300°F. Transfer rolls to rack to cool about 5 minutes. Slice each roll diagonally into 20 (1/2-inch) slices. Place cut side down on cookie sheets. Bake for 6 to 8 minutes. Turn cookies over and bake an additional 6 to 8 minutes or until dry. Remove cookies to wire rack to cool. Store in a covered container.

CHOCOLATE JAM THUMBPRINTS

DON'T WAIT FOR HOLIDAY BAKING TO MAKE THESE, THEY ARE SO GOOD
Prep time: 20 min   Bake time: 12 min
Makes: 60   Serving size: 2 Cookies
Exchanges: 1 Starch (1 Carbohydrate Choice)
Analysis per serving: 86 Calories, 16 g Carbohydrate, 2 g Protein,
2 g Fat, 11 mg Cholesterol, 60 mg Sodium, 1 g Fiber

1	cup whole-wheat flour
2	cups all-purpose flour
1/4	cup cocoa
1	tsp baking soda
1/2	cup (1 stick) light butter or light margarine, softened
1/2	cup sugar
3	large egg whites
1	large egg
1	tsp vanilla
1/2	cup low-sugar berry jam of your choice

Sift flours, cocoa and baking soda onto a piece of waxed paper or into a small bowl; set aside.

In medium bowl, use an electric mixer to beat light butter at high speed. Scrape sides of bowl with rubber spatula and gradually beat in sugar at medium speed, scraping sides occasionally, until mixture is fluffy. Add egg whites, egg and vanilla; beat at medium speed until well blended.

Use rubber spatula to scrape sides of bowl and clean beaters. Use the spatula to gently stir flour mixture into butter mixture until blended. Remove batter from bowl and wrap in plastic wrap. Chill at least 1 hour.

Preheat oven 350°F. Spray baking sheets with cooking spray.

Use floured hands to roll about 1 tablespoon of dough into a ball. Place each ball 1-inch apart on prepared baking sheet. When baking sheet is filled, use your thumb to press an indentation into center of each cookie. Each cookie should spread to about 1 1/2 inches. Bake for 8 minutes. Remove baking sheet from oven and spoon jam into each cookie indentation. Return cookies to oven and bake about 4 more minutes or until browned. Immediately use a metal spatula to remove baked cookies to a rack to cool. Proceed with remaining dough. When cookies are cool, place in container with waxed paper between layers. Store tightly covered or freeze.

EASY APPLE BARS

GRANNY SMITH APPLES ARE PERFECT FOR THIS RECIPE
Prep time: 20 min   Bake time: 45 min
Makes: 16   Serving size: 1 Bar, 1/16 Portion
Exchanges: 1 Fruit and 1 Fat (1 Carbohydrate Choice)
Analysis per serving: 96 Calories, 11 g Carbohydrate, 2 g Protein,
5 g Fat, 13 mg Cholesterol, 51 mg Sodium, 1 g Fiber

1/3	cup chopped pecans
2	cups peeled, chopped tart apples (2 medium)
1/4	cup sugar
1/2	cup whole-wheat flour
1/2	cup all-purpose flour
1	tsp cinnamon
1/2	tsp baking powder
1/2	tsp baking soda
1/4	cup cold, strong coffee
1/4	cup olive or canola oil
1	large egg or 1/4 cup egg substitute
1	tsp vanilla

Preheat oven to 350°F. Place nuts on baking sheet; bake 3 to 5 minutes
or until toasted; set aside.

In an 8- or 9-inch baking pan, spread chopped apples and sprinkle with
sugar. Let stand 10 minutes to draw out juices. Use a fork to stir in sugar,
flours and spices until apples are coated.

Use a rubber spatula to stir in coffee, oil, egg and vanilla, scraping any
ingredients clinging to sides, corners and bottom of pan into batter, until
well mixed. Smooth top with spatula.

Bake 45 to 50 minutes or until wooden pick inserted in center of cake
comes out clean. Cool on rack. Cut into 16 squares. Store covered.
Refrigerate after 2 days or freeze.

APPLE-OAT BRAN BARS

A DELICIOUS WAY TO INCORPORATE OAT BRAN INTO YOUR DIET
Prep time: 10 min   Bake time: 20 min
Makes: 24   Serving size: 1 Bar, 1/24 Portion
Exchanges: 1/2 Fruit and 1 Fat (1 Carbohydrate Choice)
Analysis per serving: 88 Calories, 12 g Carbohydrate, 2 g Protein,
4 g Fat, 0 mg Cholesterol, 89 mg Sodium, 1 g Fiber

1/2	cup chopped nuts
1/2	cup whole-wheat flour
1/2	cup all-purpose flour
1	cup oat bran
1	tsp baking powder
1/2	tsp baking soda
1	tsp cinnamon
1/4	tsp ground cloves
1	stick (1/2 cup) light margarine or light butter
1/2	cup sugar
1/2	cup egg substitute
1	large apple, peeled, cored & coarsely grated (about 1 /12 cups)

Preheat oven to 375°F. Place nuts on baking sheet and bake 3 to 5 minutes or until toasted; set aside. Spray a 13x9x2-inch pan with cooking spray.

On waxed paper or in small bowl, combine flours, oat bran, baking powder, baking soda and spices.

In medium bowl, with electric mixer at medium speed, beat margarine and sugar until light and fluffy; scrape sides of bowl . With mixer at medium speed, add egg substitute, beating well. Scrape sides of bowl . Add combined dry ingredients and mix at low speed until well blended. Use a rubber spatula to gently mix in grated apple and toasted nuts. Spread in prepared pan.

Bake 20 to 25 minutes or until lightly brown. Cool on rack. If desired, sprinkle with confectioners' sugar. Cut into 24 squares. Store covered. Refrigerate after 2 days or freeze.

APPLE RAISIN BARS

QUICK & EASY TO MAKE
Prep time: 10 min   Bake time: 25 min
Makes: 16   Serving size: 1 Bar, 1/16 Portion
Exchanges: 1 Starch and 1 Fat (1 Carbohydrate Choice)
Analysis per serving: 117 Calories, 17 g Carbohydrate, 3 g Protein,
4 g Fat, 26 mg Cholesterol, 134 mg Sodium, 1 g Fiber

1/2	cup unsweetened applesauce
1/2	cup unsweetened apple juice
2	large eggs
2	large egg whites
1/4	cup olive or canola oil
1	cup all-purpose flour
1	cup whole-wheat flour
1	tsp baking soda
2	tsp baking powder
1	tsp nutmeg
1 1/2	tsp cinnamon
1/2	cup raisins

Preheat oven to 350°F. Spray an 8-inch square pan with cooking spray.

In medium bowl with electric mixer at medium speed, beat together applesauce, juice, eggs, egg whites and olive oil until well blended; scrape sides of bowl . Add flours, baking soda, baking powder and spices and beat at medium speed until well blended. Scrape sides and use a rubber spatula to stir in raisins.

Spoon batter into prepared pan and bake for 25 minutes or until pick inserted in center comes out clean. Cool on rack. Cut into 16 bars. Store covered. Refrigerate after 2 days or freeze up to 3 months.

GOLDEN APPLE BARS

THESE ARE VERY FRAGILE — USE A METAL SPATULA TO REMOVE FROM PAN
Prep time: 15 min   Bake time: 20 min
Makes: 50   Serving size: 1 Bar, 1/50 Portion
Exchanges: 1/2 Fruit and 1 Fat (1 Carbohydrate Choice)
Analysis per serving: 76 Calories, 9 g Carbohydrate, 2 g Protein,
4 g Fat, 5 mg Cholesterol, 20 mg Sodium, 1 g Fiber

Pastry

1	large egg or 1/4 cup egg substitute
1	cup whole-wheat flour
1	cup all-purpose flour
1/4	cup sugar
1/2	cup olive or canola oil
1	tsp vanilla extract

Spray a jelly roll pan (15x10x1-inch) with cooking spray. In a medium bowl, use a fork to beat egg. Stir in remaining ingredients; mix until well blended. Pat onto bottom of prepared pan.

Filling

5	cups Golden Delicious apples, peeled & cored (4 or 5 apples)
2	Tbs lemon juice
3	Tbs all-purpose flour
1/4	cup sugar
1	tsp cinnamon
1	tsp dried lemon peel or grated fresh lemon peel
1/4	tsp nutmeg
1	cup shredded low-fat sharp cheddar cheese

Preheat oven to 425°F. Thinly slice apples into a large bowl. Sprinkle sliced apples with lemon juice. Combine apples with remaining ingredients and spread evenly over unbaked crust. Sprinkle topping over apple mixture.

Topping

1/2	cup whole-wheat flour
1/4	cup all-purpose flour
3	Tbs brown sugar
1/4	cup olive or canola oil

Use a fork to combine all ingredients until crumbly. Sprinkle evenly over apple filling. Bake 20 to 25 minutes or until apples are tender and topping is browned. Cut into dessert-sized portions or cookie bars.

CHOCOLATE JAM SQUARES

COMES WITH ITS OWN FROSTING
Prep time: 10 min   Bake time: 10 min
Makes: 16   Serving size: 1 Bar, 1/16 Portion
Exchanges: 1 Fruit (1 Carbohydrate Choice)
Analysis per serving: 68 Calories, 11 g Carbohydrate, 1 g Protein,
3 g Fat, 0 mg Cholesterol, 35 mg Sodium, 1 g Fiber

1/2	cup all-purpose flour
1/4	cup whole-wheat flour
1/3	cup sugar
1/2	tsp baking soda
3	Tbs cocoa
1/2	cup water
1	tsp vanilla
3	Tbs white vinegar
3	Tbs olive or canola oil
3	Tbs low-sugar raspberry or strawberry jam

Preheat oven 375°F. Spray an 8-inch square baking pan with cooking spray.

In medium bowl, using a wooden spoon or rubber spatula, combine flours, sugar, baking soda and cocoa.

Measure 1/2 cup water in 1-cup glass measuring cup and microwave on High for 1 1/2 minutes. Stir in vanilla, vinegar and oil. Stir into dry ingredients and combine until well mixed.

Spoon into prepared pan. Bake 10 minutes.

Three minutes before cake is done baking, place jam in same glass measuring cup. Microwave 30 seconds. Stir.

Remove cake from oven and immediately spread warmed jam over baked cake. Cool on rack. When cool, cut into 16 bars.

SIMPLE BANANA NUT BARS

TO USE UP RIPE BANANAS — MADE IN THE SAME PAN IN WHICH IT'S BAKED
Prep Time: 10 min   Bake time: 30 min
Makes: 16   Serving size: 1 Bar, 1/16 Portion
Exchanges: 1 Starch and 1 Fat (1 Carbohydrate Choice)
Analysis per serving: 124 Calories, 16 g Carbohydrate, 3 g Protein,
6 g Fat, 0 mg Cholesterol, 62 mg Sodium, 1 g Fiber

1/4	cup chopped nuts
3/4	cup whole-wheat flour
3/4	cup all-purpose flour
1/4	cup sugar
1	tsp baking powder
1/4	tsp baking soda
1/2	tsp cinnamon
1/4	tsp nutmeg
1	cup very ripe bananas, mashed (2 medium)
1/3	cup olive or canola oil
1/3	cup buttermilk
1/2	cup egg substitute

Preheat oven to 350°F. Have an 8- or 9-inch square pan ready. Place nuts on baking sheet; bake about 3 to 5 minutes or until browned; set aside.

Put flours, sugar, baking powder, baking soda and spices into pan and stir with fork to mix well. Stir in mashed bananas, oil, buttermilk, egg substitute and toasted nuts and mix until blended. Use a rubber spatula to scrape any ingredients clinging to sides, corners or bottom of pan into batter.

Bake 30 to 35 minutes or until lightly browned and wooden pick inserted in center comes out clean. Cool on rack. Cut into 16 squares. Store covered. Refrigerate after 2 days or freeze.

BANANA POPPY SEED BARS

A FAVORITE COOKIE BAR FOR BANANA LOVERS
Prep time: 15 min   Bake time: 25 min
Makes: 16   Serving size: 1 Bar, 1/16 Portion
Exchanges: 1 Starch and 1/2 Fat (1 Carbohydrate Choice)
Analysis per serving: 94 Calories, 15 g Carbohydrate, 2 g Protein,
3 g Fat, 13 mg Cholesterol, 78 mg Sodium, 1 g Fiber

1	cup whole-wheat flour
2/3	cup all-purpose flour
1	tsp baking soda
1/4	cup sugar
1	Tbs poppy seeds

Preheat oven to 375°F. Spray 8-inch square pan with cooking spray.

In medium bowl, use a rubber spatula to mix all ingredients. Make a well in bowl and add the following ingredients to the well. Use the spatula to thoroughly combine.

1	ripe banana, mashed (1/2 cup)
1	tsp dried lemon peel or grated fresh lemon peel
3/4	cup skim milk
3	Tbs olive or canola oil
3	Tbs lemon juice
1	large egg, beaten or 1/4 cup egg substitute

Spoon batter into prepared baking pan. Bake 25 minutes or until lightly browned and when a pick inserted in center, comes out clean. Cool on rack. Cut into 16 squares. Store covered. Refrigerate after 2 days or freeze.

QUICK CARROT BARS

TO SAVE TIME, USE RAW BABY CARROTS — NO NEED TO PEEL OR SLICE
Prep time: 10 min   Bake time: 35 min
Makes: 24   Serving size: 1 Bar, 1/24 Portion
Exchanges: 1/2 Starch and 1 Fat (1 Carbohydrate Choice)
Analysis per serving: 101 Calories, 10 g Carbohydrate, 2 g Protein,
6 g Fat, 0 mg Cholesterol, 22 mg Sodium, 1 g Fiber

1/2	cup chopped walnuts
1	cup whole-wheat flour
1/2	cup all-purpose flour
1/2	tsp baking powder
1/2	tsp cinnamon
1/2	cup coconut (optional)
1/2	cup olive or canola oil
1/4	cup unsweetened applesauce
1/2	cup brown sugar
1/2	cup egg substitute
2	cups 1/2-inch thick-sliced carrots

Preheat oven to 350°F. Place chopped nuts on baking sheet and bake for about 5 minutes or until browned; set aside. Spray a 13x9x2-inch pan with cooking spray.

In medium bowl, combine flours, baking powder, cinnamon and coconut (if using).

In food processor, process oil, applesauce, sugar and egg substitute until blended; scrape sides. With machine running, gradually add carrot slices until coarsely chopped. Use a rubber spatula to stir carrot mixture and toasted nuts into flour mixture until well mixed. Spread into prepared pan.

Bake 35 minutes or until edges pull away from sides and top browns slightly. Cool on rack. Cut into 24 bars. If desired, sprinkle with confectioners' sugar or frost with LIGHT CREAM CHEESE FROSTING (page 78) Store covered.

CHEWY COCONUT SQUARES

THESE BARS ARE LIKE COFFEE CAKE
Prep time: 10 min   Bake time: 35 min
Makes: 16   Serving size: 1 Square, 1/16 Portion
Exchanges: 1/2 Fruit and 1 Fat (1 Carbohydrate Choice)
Analysis per serving: 68 Calories, 7 g Carbohydrate, 1 g Protein,
4 g Fat, 17 mg Cholesterol, 25 mg Sodium, 1 g Fiber

1/3	cup chopped nuts
1/4	cup light butter or light margarine, softened
4	Tbs sugar, divided
1/2	cup whole-wheat flour
2	Tbs all-purpose flour
1	large egg or 1/4 cup egg substitute
1	tsp vanilla extract
1/2	cup shredded coconut

Preheat oven to 350°F. Place chopped nuts on baking sheet; bake 3 to 5 minutes or until toasted; set aside. Spray an 8-inch square pan with cooking spray.

In medium bowl, cream light butter and 2 Tbs sugar with electric mixer at medium speed until light and fluffy. With mixer at low speed, blend in flours. Scrape sides of bowl and turn batter into prepared pan, spreading evenly. Bake 10 minutes.

In same bowl, combine toasted nuts, egg, vanilla and coconut until well blended. Spread evenly over baked dough. Bake 25 minutes or until golden. While warm cut into 16 squares. Cool on rack.   Store covered.

CHOCOLATE CRUNCH BARS

IF YOU LIKE REESE'S PIECES®, YOU'LL LOVE THESE BARS
Prep time: 10 min   Cook time: 1 hr
Serves: 16   Serving size: 1 Bar, 1/16 Portion
Exchanges: 1 Starch and 1 Fat (1 Carbohydrate Choice)
Analysis per serving: 128 Calories, 15 g Carbohydrate, 5 g Protein,
6 g Fat, 0 mg Cholesterol, 17 mg Sodium, 1 g Fiber

3 1/2	**cups toasted natural brown rice cereal**
3/4	**cup natural peanut butter**
2	**medium bananas, thinly sliced**
1	**recipe FABULOUS CHOCOLATE PUDDING (page 188), prepared**

Spray a 9-inch pan with cooking spray; set aside.

Spray a large bowl with cooking spray and put in peanut butter. Microwave on High for 1 minute. Spray a rubber spatula with cooking spray and stir in cereal until cereal is coated with peanut butter. Use the spatula to press half of mixture into prepared pan. Layer sliced bananas over cereal mixture.

Pour pudding over bananas. Gently press remaining cereal mixture onto pudding. Chill at least 1 hour or until firm enough to cut into 16 squares.

❖ Grainfields® toasted natural brown rice cereal or Kashi® puffed cereal are suggested. Most large food stores or health food stores carry such cereals

DEVILISHLY DELICIOUS CHOCOLATE BARS

SO MOIST AND TASTY!
Prep time: 10 min   Bake time: 30 min
Makes: 24   Serving size: 1 Bar, 1/24 Portion
Exchanges: 1 Fruit (1 Carbohydrate Choice)
Analysis per serving: 68 Calories, 12 g Carbohydrate, 2 g Protein,
1 g Fat, 0 mg Cholesterol, 114 mg Sodium, 1 g Fiber

1/2	**cup unsweetened applesauce**
1/2	**cup sugar**
1	**tsp vanilla extract**
2	**Tbs olive or canola oil**
1/2	**cup egg substitute**
1	**cup whole-wheat flour**
1	**cup all-purpose flour**
1/4	**cup cocoa**
1/4	**tsp salt**
1	**cup buttermilk**
1 1/2	**tsp baking soda**
1	**Tbs white vinegar**

Preheat oven 350°F. Spray 13x9x2-inch baking pan with cooking spray.

In large bowl, with electric mixer at medium speed, beat applesauce, sugar, vanilla and oil until well blended; scrape sides of bowl. Add egg substitute and beat at medium speed until blended; scrape sides of bowl.

In small bowl, combine flours, cocoa and salt. With mixer at medium speed, alternately add flour mixture and buttermilk to creamed mixture beginning and ending with flour mixture until well mixed. Scrape sides of bowl after each addition.

In custard cup, combine baking soda and white vinegar until blended. Using a rubber spatula, carefully fold vinegar mixture into batter (do not use mixer) until blended. Spoon into prepared pan and bake 30 to 35 minutes or until pick inserted in center of cake comes out clean. Cool on rack for 15 minutes before cutting into 24 squares.

❖ To make Cherry or Strawberry Chocolate Squares, reduce vanilla extract to 1/2 tsp and add 2 tsp cherry or strawberry extract to applesauce mixture. Proceed as directed.

MIX-IN-THE-PAN DATE BARS

MIX AND BAKE IN THE SAME PAN FOR A FAST FIXING SNACK BAR
Prep time: 5 min   Bake time: 30 min.
Makes: 16   Serving size: 1 Bar, 1/16 Portion
Exchanges: 1 Fruit and 1 Fat (1 Carbohydrate Choice)
Analysis per serving: 107 Calories, 15 g Carbohydrate, 2 g Protein,
5 g Fat, 0 mg Cholesterol, 27 mg Sodium, 2 g Fiber

1/4	cup chopped nuts
1/2	cup whole-wheat flour
1/2	cup all-purpose flour
1/2	tsp nutmeg
1/2	tsp baking powder
2	Tbs sugar
1/4	cup olive or canola oil
1/2	cup egg substitute
1	Tbs lemon juice
1	cup chopped dates

Preheat oven to 350°F. Place nuts on baking sheet; bake 3 to 5 minutes or until browned; set aside.

In a 9-inch square pan, mix flours, nutmeg, baking powder and sugar. Add oil, egg substitute and lemon juice. With rubber spatula, mix and stir until well blended. Stir in dates and toasted nuts.

Bake about 30 minutes or until lightly browned and toothpick inserted in center comes out clean. Cool in pan on rack. Cut into 16 bars. Store covered.

DATE CHEWS

CHEWY LITTLE GOODIES
Prep time: 5 min   Bake time: 20 min
Makes: 16   Serving size: 1 Piece, 1/16 Portion
Exchanges: 1 Fruit (1 Carbohydrate Choice)
Analysis per serving: 68 Calories, 12 g Carbohydrate, 1 g Protein,
2 g Fat, 13 mg Cholesterol, 17 mg Sodium, 1 g Fiber

2	Tbs sugar
1	cup chopped dates
1/4	cup whole-wheat flour
1/4	cup all-purpose flour
1/2	tsp baking powder
2	Tbs olive or canola oil
1	large egg, beaten or 1/4 cup egg substitute

Preheat oven to 350°F. Spray a 9-inch square pan with cooking spray.

In medium bowl, combine sugar, dates, flours and baking powder. Use a rubber spatula to stir in oil and egg until well mixed. Dough will be very thick. Spread evenly with spatula into prepared pan.

Bake 20 minutes or until lightly browned or pick inserted in center comes out clean. While warm cut into 16 squares. Cool in pan on rack. These bars do not rise. If desired, sprinkle with confectioners' sugar. Store covered.

GINGERBREAD BARS

AN OLD FAVORITE MADE THE LOW-FAT WAY
Prep time: 10 min   Bake time: 30 min
Makes: 16   Serving size: 1 Bar, 1/16 Portion
Exchanges: 1/2 Starch and 1/2 Fat (1 Carbohydrate Choice)
Analysis per serving: 65 Calories, 10 g Carbohydrate, 2 g Protein,
2 g Fat, 13 mg Cholesterol, 88 mg Sodium, 1 g Fiber

1/2	cup whole-wheat flour
1/2	cup all-purpose flour
1/2	tsp baking soda
1/4	tsp salt
1	tsp cinnamon
1 1/2	tsp ginger
1/8	tsp ground cloves
1	large egg
2	Tbs brown sugar
1/4	cup molasses
1/2	cup buttermilk
2	Tbs olive or canola oil

Preheat oven to 350°F. Spray an 8-inch square pan with cooking spray.

Sift flours, baking soda, salt and spices onto waxed paper or into small bowl.

In medium bowl, beat egg, sugar and molasses with electric mixer at medium speed until light. Scrape sides of bowl. Add buttermilk, oil and reserved flour mixture and beat at medium speed until smooth, scraping bowl occasionally.

Spoon into prepared pan and bake 30 minutes or until pick inserted in center comes out clean. Cool on rack. Cut into 16 pieces.

PUMPKIN PIE SQUARES

PUMPKIN PIE LOVERS, HERE'S A VARIATION!
Prep time: 20 min   Bake time: 50 min
Makes: 16   Serving size: 1 Bar, 1/16 Portion
Exchanges: 1 Starch and 1 Fat (1 Carbohydrate Choice)
Analysis per serving: 131 Calories, 16 g Carbohydrate, 5 g Protein,
6 g Fat, 1 mg Cholesterol, 81 mg Sodium, 2 g Fiber

1/2	**cup whole-wheat flour**
1/2	**cup all-purpose flour**
1/2	**cup old-fashioned oats**
5	**Tbs brown sugar, divided**
1/3	**cup olive or canola oil**
1/2	**cup egg substitute**
1	**12-ounce can evaporated skim milk**
2	**cups cooked pumpkin or 1 16-ounce can natural pumpkin (NOT pie filling)**
1	**Tbs pumpkin pie spice**
1/4	**tsp salt**
1/4	**cup chopped walnuts**

Preheat oven to 350°F. Spray 9-inch square pan with cooking spray.

In medium bowl, use a rubber spatula to combine flours, oatmeal and 2 Tbs brown sugar. Add oil and mix until blended. Press 1 cup of mixture onto pan bottom; reserve remainder. Bake about 10 minutes or until browned.

Meanwhile, in medium bowl, using a whisk, beat egg substitute. Shake evaporated milk and add to egg substitute along with pumpkin and remaining 3 Tbs brown sugar, spice and salt; beat with whisk until well blended; pour over baked crust. Bake 30 minutes.

Mix reserved flour mixture with chopped nuts and sprinkle over pumpkin filling. Bake 10 minutes longer or until filling is set and top lightly browned. Cool in pan on rack. When cool, refrigerate at least 1 hour before cutting into 16 squares. Store, covered, in refrigerator.

RAISIN SPICE SQUARES

THE RAISINS CONTRIBUTE SWEETNESS, MOISTURE, TEXTURE AND FLAVOR
Prep time: 15 min   Bake time: 25 min
Makes: 24   Serving size: 1 Bar, 1/24 Portion
Exchanges: 1/2 Starch and 1 Fat (1 Carbohydrate Choice)
Analysis per serving: 85 Calories, 12 g Carbohydrate, 2 g Protein,
4 g Fat, 9 mg Cholesterol, 74 mg Sodium, 1 g Fiber

1/3	cup chopped walnuts
1	cup whole-wheat flour
1	cup all-purpose flour
1	tsp baking soda
1	tsp cinnamon
1	tsp nutmeg
1/4	tsp salt
1/2	cup raisins
2	cups water
1	large egg or 1/4 cup egg substitute
1/4	cup olive or canola oil
1/4	cup unsweetened applesauce
1/4	cup sugar

Preheat oven to 350°F. Place chopped nuts on baking sheet; bake 3 to 5 minutes or until toasted; set aside. Spray a 13x9x2-inch pan with cooking spray.

Sift flours, baking soda, cinnamon, nutmeg and salt into a large bowl. If grains remain in sifter, just add to dry ingredients; stir in toasted nuts.

In a 4-cup glass measuring cup, combine raisins and water. Microwave on High for 10 minutes, stirring after 5 minutes. Remove from microwave; stir and cool to lukewarm. Use a rubber spatula to stir in egg until well mixed. Stir in oil, applesauce and sugar until blended.

Pour raisin mixture into flour mixture and mix until thoroughly combined. Scrape sides of bowl and spoon batter into prepared pan.

Bake for 25 minutes or until wooden pick inserted in center comes out clean. Cool on wire rack. Cut into 24 squares or bars. If desired, sprinkle with confectioners' sugar. Store covered.

RASPBERRY BARS

YOU CAN SUBSTITUTE YOUR FAVORITE JAM
Prep time: 10 min   Bake time: 35 min
Makes: 16   Serving size: 1 Bar, 1/16 Portion
Exchanges: 1 Starch and 1 Fat (1 Carbohydrate Choice)
Analysis per serving: 116 Calories, 17 g Carbohydrate, 2 g Protein,
5 g Fat, 0 mg Cholesterol, 20 mg Sodium, 1 g Fiber

1/2	cup whole-wheat flour
1/2	cup all-purpose flour
1	cup old-fashioned oats
1/4	tsp baking soda
2	Tbs light brown sugar
1/3	cup olive or canola oil
2/3	cup low-sugar raspberry jam

Preheat oven to 350°F. Spray an 8-inch square pan with cooking spray. Line with aluminum foil and spray again.

In medium bowl, combine flours, oatmeal, baking soda, brown sugar and oil.   Press 1 cup of mixture onto bottom of prepared pan. Spread jam to within 1/4 inch of the edge. Sprinkle reserved crumb mixture over top and lightly press into the jam.

Bake 35 to 40 minutes. Cool on rack. Remove baked cookies with aluminum foil from pan and place on cutting board. Use a sharp knife to cut into 24 bars.   Use a metal spatula to remove bars from aluminum foil. Store covered.

TANGY CITRUS BARS

CRANBERRIES GIVE THESE MOIST BARS A TANGY FLAVOR
Prep time: 10 min   Bake time: 35 min
Makes: 24   Serving size: 1 Bar, 1/24 Portion
Exchanges: 1/2 Starch and 1 Fat (1 Carbohydrate Choice)
Analysis per serving: 91 Calories, 12 g Carbohydrate, 2 g Protein,
4 g Fat, 0 mg Cholesterol, 93 mg Sodium, 1 g Fiber

1/3	cup chopped nuts
1/2	cup egg substitute
1/4	cup olive or canola oil
1 1/2	cups orange juice
1/2	tsp orange extract
1 1/2	cups whole-wheat flour
1/2	tsp cinnamon
1/2	tsp nutmeg
1 1/2	cups whole or chopped cranberries

Preheat oven 350°F. Place chopped nuts on baking sheet; bake 3 to 5 minutes or until toasted; set aside. Spray 13x9x2-inch pan with cooking spray.

In medium bowl with electric mixer at medium speed, beat egg substitute, oil, juice and extract until well mixed; scrape sides of bowl. Add flour and spices and beat at low speed, scraping sides of bowl, until dry ingredients are incorporated. Use a rubber spatula to stir in cranberries and toasted nuts. Spoon mixture into prepared pan; sprinkle with topping.

Topping

1/2	cup all-purpose flour
1	tsp baking soda
2	tsp baking powder
1/2	cup flaked coconut
1	8-ounce can juice-packed crushed pineapple, drained

In same bowl, combine all topping ingredients until well mixed. Reserve pineapple juice for another use.

Bake 35 to 40 minutes or until browned and pick inserted in center comes out clean. Cool on rack. Cut into 24 bars or squares. Store covered. Refrigerate after 2 days.

FANTASTIC FUDGEY BROWNIES

VERY RICH BUT GREAT WHEN FROZEN AND DEFROSTED
Prep time: 10 min   Bake time: 20 min
Makes: 48   Serving Size: 1 Brownie, 1/48 Portion
Exchanges: 1/2 Starch and 1/2 Fat (1 Carbohydrate Choice)
Analysis per serving: 61 Calories, 9 Carbohydrate, 1 g Protein,
3 g Fat, 3 mg Cholesterol, 39 mg Sodium, 1 g Fiber (without nuts)

1/2	cup chopped nuts (optional)
1/2	cup light butter or light margarine
2	squares (1 ounce each) unsweetened chocolate
1	cup reduced-fat chocolate chips (or 1/2 cup mini chips)
3/4	cup whole-wheat flour
3/4	cup all-purpose flour
1/2	cup unsweetened applesauce
1	tsp baking powder (omit if nuts are used)
1	cup egg substitute
1/2	cup sugar
1	tsp vanilla

Preheat oven to 325°F. If using nuts, place on baking sheet; bake 3-5 minutes or until toasted; set aside. Spray a 13x9x2-inch baking pan with cooking spray.

In a glass 4-cup measuring cup, put light butter, chocolate squares and chips. Microwave on High for 2 minutes; stir. Microwave 1 minute more or until mixture is smooth. Stir in flours, applesauce and baking powder until well blended; cool.

In a large bowl with electric mixer at medium speed, beat egg substitute, sugar and vanilla for 3 minutes, scraping bowl occasionally. Add chocolate mixture to egg mixture and beat at low speed until well blended, about 30 seconds, scraping bowl to incorporate all ingredients. Using a rubber spatula, stir in chopped nuts.

Spoon batter into prepared pan and bake 25 to 28 minutes or until pick inserted in center comes out clean. Do not overbake. Cool on wire rack.

When cool, cut into 24 squares. Store in a covered container for no more than 2 days at room temperature or freeze up to 3 months. If frozen, defrost before serving.

Cakes

Chiffon, Angel Food and Sponge Cakes are light and delicate and are easy to modify. Chiffon cake combines beaten egg whites, egg yolks, leavening and a small amount of oil. Angel food cake has no leavening, no shortening and no egg yolks; therefore, no cholesterol and no fat. It can be baked in a tube pan or loaf pan. Sponge cake uses both egg whites and egg yolks, with no fat added. Sponge cake may also be used as a roll cake.

Bake tube cake in tube pan on bottom rack in oven.

Do not open oven door until minimum baking time has elapsed.

Cakes baked in a tube pan are done when cracks in top feel dry and no imprint remains when top is lightly touched. Foam-type cakes baked in oblong or jelly roll pans are done when a wooden pick inserted in center comes out clean.

To remove cooled cake from tube pan, loosen first by moving a knife up and down against sides and center tube of pan. Turn cake upside down and remove pan.

A filled carbonated beverage bottle makes a convenient stand for a tube or bundt pan that must be inverted to cool.

Whole-wheat flour should be stirred with a fork before measuring to ensure a light-textured baked good. When sifting whole-wheat flour, bran particles will remain in sifter. Just add them to the batter along with the sifted flour. Whole-wheat pastry flour can be substituted for whole-wheat flour in baked goods. The texture of the cake, cookies or pie crusts will be lighter. Whole-wheat pastry flour is preferred if available.

Use white whole-wheat flour if available in place of darker whole-wheat flour. Its texture and color is lighter, but it does have all the nutrients and fiber of regular whole-wheat flour. Many large food stores do carry it under the King Arthur name in the baking aisle. If you prefer to use only white all-purpose flour, do so. I prefer combining all-purpose flour and whole-wheat flour because whole-wheat flour has natural nutrients and fiber. By combining both flours, we get a healthy baked good that is tasty.

RASPBERRY ANGEL FOOD CAKE

MY FAMILY'S FAVORITE CAKE
Prep time: 10 min   Bake time: 40 min
Serves: 16   Serving size: 1 Slice, 1/16 Portion
Exchanges: 1 Starch (1 Carbohydrate Choice)
Meat Analysis per serving: 66 Calories, 14 g Carbohydrates, 3 g Protein,
0 Fat, 0 Cholesterol, 34 mg Sodium, 1 g Fiber

10	**large egg whites, at room temperature**
1 1/4	**tsp cream of tartar**
1	**tsp vanilla extract**
1/2	**tsp almond extract**
1/2	**cup sugar**
1	**cup cake flour**
2	**cups fresh raspberries, washed & well drained**

Preheat oven to 325°F. Have an ungreased 10-inch tube pan ready. In large bowl, beat egg whites at high speed until frothy; beat in cream of tartar until soft peaks form. Add extracts and gradually beat in sugar at high speed, scraping bowl occasionally. Beat until whites are stiff but not dry when lifted with a rubber spatula.

Sift flour over beaten whites and sprinkle berries over sifted flour in bowl. Use a rubber spatula to gently fold flour and raspberries into batter. Thoroughly mix to incorporate all flour. Spoon mixture into pan, gently cut through batter with a clean knife and level top.

Bake 40 to 45 minutes or until lightly browned and pick inserted in center comes out clean. Immediately invert over a sturdy bottle or funnel and cool completely, about 1 hour. Use a knife to loosen cake from sides, center tube and bottom of pan; remove cake and place on plate. Store covered at room temperature for up to 2 days. Can be frozen up to 3 months.

Use a serrated knife for easy slicing.

ORANGE CHIFFON CAKE

A DELICATE, LIGHT CAKE THAT SERVES BEAUTIFULLY WITH FRUIT
Prep time: 10 min   Bake time: 55 min
Serves: 16   Serving size: 1 Slice, 1/16 Portion
Exchanges: 1 Starch and 1/2 Fat (1 Carbohydrate Choice)
Analysis per serving: 100 Calories, 14 g Carbohydrates, 5 g Protein,
3 g Fat, 107 mg Cholesterol, 180 mg Sodium, 0 g Fiber

8	large egg whites, at room temperature
1/2	tsp cream of tartar
2 1/4	cups sifted cake flour
1/2	cup sugar, divided
1	Tbs baking powder
1/2	tsp salt
1/2	cup olive or canola oil
4	large egg yolks, at room temperature
3/4	cup orange juice
1	tsp vanilla extract
2	Tbs dried orange peel or grated fresh orange peel

Preheat oven to 325°F. Have an ungreased 10-inch tube pan ready.

In large bowl, beat egg whites with electric mixer at high speed until frothy. Add cream of tartar and continue beating at high speed until soft peaks form. Gradually beat 1/4 cup sugar into whites at high speed, scraping sides of bowl occasionally, until whites are stiff when beaters are lifted. Set aside.

In another large bowl, sift sifted flour, remaining 1/4 cup sugar, baking powder and salt. Make a well and add: oil, yolks, juice, extract and peel; beat on medium speed until smooth, about 30 seconds, scraping sides of bowl occasionally. Pour flour mixture over beaten whites and gently fold whites into batter just until blended and no white streaks remain. Spoon into pan and bake 55 minutes or until pick inserted in center comes out clean and cake springs back when touched lightly.

Immediately invert cake over a sturdy bottle or funnel and cool completely, about 1 hour. When cool, use a knife to loosen sides, center tube and bottom of cake from pan. Remove cake and place on plate. Store covered. Can be frozen up to 3 months.

Use a serrated knife for easy slicing.

ISLAND CHIFFON CAKE

RIPE BANANAS AND PINEAPPLE JUICE MAKE THIS CAKE A TUMMY PLEASER
Prep time: 10 min   Bake time: 55 min
Serves: 16   Serving size: 1 Slice, 1/16 Portion
Exchanges: 1 Starch, 1/2 Fruit and 2 Fat (2 Carbohydrate Choices)
Analysis per serving: 201 Calories, 24 g Carbohydrates, 5 g Protein,
10 g Fat, 107 mg Cholesterol, 180 mg Sodium, 2 g Fiber

1	**cup (7 or 8) large egg whites, at room temperature**
1/2	**tsp cream of tartar**
1/4	**cup sugar**

Preheat oven to 325°F. Have an ungreased 10-inch tube pan ready.

In a large bowl, beat egg whites with electric mixer at high speed until frothy; beat in cream of tartar. Gradually add sugar, beating at high speed and scraping bowl often, until stiff peaks are formed when lifted with a rubber spatula. Set aside.

In another large bowl, sift the following ingredients together and make a well.

1	**cup and 3 Tbs whole-wheat flour**
1	**cup all-purpose flour**
1/4	**cup sugar**
1/2	**tsp salt**
1	**Tbs baking powder**
1/2	**tsp cinnamon**
1/4	**tsp nutmeg**
1	**tsp dried lemon peel or grated fresh lemon peel**

Add the following ingredients to the well in order listed:

1/2	**cup olive or canola oil**
1	**cup mashed ripe bananas (2 medium)**
4	**egg yolks**
1	**6-ounce can (3/4 cup) unsweetened pineapple juice**

Using same beaters, beat all ingredients at medium speed until smooth, scraping bowl occasionally. Slowly pour egg yolk mixture over entire surface of egg whites. Use a rubber spatula to gently fold batters just until blended and no white streaks remain. To fold, use a flexible spatula. Slip it down side of bowl to bottom; turn bowl a quarter turn and lift spatula through mixture along side of bowl with spatula parallel to surface. Turn spatula over so as to fold batter across surface. Continue until batter is blended to desired consistency. Turn batter into ungreased tube pan and bake for 55 minutes or until browned and cake springs back when touched.

Remove from oven and immediately invert over a sturdy bottle or funnel to cool. When completely cool, about 1 hour, loosen sides, center tube and bottom of cake from pan with a knife and place cake on plate. If desired, sprinkle with confectioners' sugar.

Store covered at room temperature for no more than 2 days. Can be frozen up to 3 months. Refer to pages 237-238 for wrapping suggestions and storage tips for freezing.

NUTTY MAPLE CHIFFON CAKE

A LIGHT, FLAVORFUL CAKE WITH A BIT OF CRUNCH
Prep time: 10 min   Bake time: 55 min
Serves: 16   Serving size: 1 Slice, 1/16 Portion
Exchanges: 1 Starch, 1/2 Fruit and 2 Fat (1 Carbohydrate Choice)
Analysis per serving: 213 Calories, 20 g Carbohydrate, 5 g Protein,
13 g Fat, 66 mg Cholesterol, 182 Sodium, 2 g Fiber

1	cup finely chopped pecans or walnuts
8	large egg whites, at room temperature
1/2	tsp cream of tartar
1/3	cup sugar
1	cup whole-wheat flour
1	cup all-purpose flour
1/3	cup packed brown sugar
1	Tbs baking powder
1/2	tsp salt
1/2	cup olive or canola oil
5	large egg yolks, at room temperature
3/4	cup cold water
2	tsp maple extract

Preheat oven 325°F. Place nuts on baking sheet; bake 3 to 5 minutes or until toasted; set aside. Have an ungreased 10-inch tube pan ready.

In a large bowl, use electric mixer at high speed to beat egg whites until frothy. Add cream of tartar and gradually beat in white sugar at high speed until stiff peaks form; scraping sides of bowl occasionally; set aside.

Sift flours, brown sugar, baking powder and salt into a large bowl. Make a well and add oil, yolks, water and extract. Beat with a wooden spoon until smooth. Pour flour mixture over stiffly beaten whites. Using a rubber spatula, gently fold whites into batter until no white streaks remain. Fold in toasted nuts.

Spoon into pan and bake 55 to 65 minutes or until pick inserted in center comes out clean. Immediately invert over a bottle or funnel and cool completely, about 1 hour. Loosen sides, center tube and bottom of cake from pan with a knife; place cake on a plate. Store covered. Freeze up to 3 months.

Use a serrated knife for easy slicing.

FEATHERWEIGHT SPONGE CAKE

FILL & FROST WITH TEMPTING BLUEBERRY TOPPING (page 81)
Prep time: 15 min   Bake time: 25 min
Makes: 2 8-inch layers   Serving size: 1 Slice, 1/12 Portion
Exchanges: 1 Starch (1 Carbohydrate Choice)
Analysis per serving: 74 Calories, 13 g Carbohydrate, 2 g Protein,
1 g Fat, 53 mg Cholesterol, 66 mg Sodium, 0 Fiber

3	large eggs, separated and at room temperature
1/2	cup confectioners' sugar
1/4	cup boiling water
1/2	tsp dried orange peel or grated fresh orange peel
1 1/2	tsp vanilla extract
1	cup cake flour
1 1/2	tsp baking powder

Preheat oven to 350°F. Place one 8-inch cake pan on two sheets of wax paper. Trace pan; cut wax paper into two circles. Spray both 8-inch cake pans with cooking spray; place wax paper circle on bottom of each pan; spray paper with cooking spray. Cakes will be easier to remove from pan.

In large bowl, with electric mixer at high speed, beat egg whites until stiff; set aside.

In another large bowl, with same beaters, beat egg yolks at medium speed until lemon colored; add sugar and beat at medium speed until thick and smooth, scraping sides of bowl occasionally. Add boiling water, orange peel and vanilla and beat at medium speed to combine; scrape bowl.

In small bowl, stir flour and baking powder together. Beat flour mixture into yolk mixture at medium speed a little at a time, mixing well and scraping sides of bowl after each addition, until smooth. Gently fold yolk mixture into beaten whites until no white streaks remain.

Divide batter evenly into prepared pans and bake 25 minutes or until lightly browned and pick inserted in center comes out clean. Cool on rack for 10 minutes. Use a knife to loosen cakes; remove from pans and cool completely on rack, about 30 minutes. Peel off wax paper; fill and frost as desired. Can be frozen without filling and frosting up to 3 months.

Use a serrated knife for easy slicing.

SIMPLE APPLE CAKE

SIMPLY APPLELICIOUS!
Prep time: 5 min   Bake time: 30 min
Serves: 9   Serving size: 1 Slice, 1/9 Portion
Exchanges: 1 Starch and 2 1/2 Fat (1 Carbohydrate Choice)
Analysis per serving: 172 Calories, 18 g Carbohydrate, 3 g Protein,
10 g Fat, 0 mg Cholesterol, 87 mg Sodium, 2 g Fiber

1/4	cup chopped nuts
1/3	cup whole-wheat flour
1/2	cup all-purpose flour
1/4	cup brown sugar
1/2	tsp baking soda
1/2	tsp cinnamon
1/3	cup olive or canola oil
1/2	cup egg substitute
1	tsp vanilla extract
2	cups peeled, chopped apples (2 medium)

Preheat oven to 350°F. Place chopped nuts on baking sheet; bake 3 to 5 minutes or until toasted; set aside. Spray a 9-inch square cake pan with cooking spray.

In large bowl, use electric mixer at low speed to beat flours, brown sugar, baking soda, cinnamon, oil, egg substitute and extract for 1 minute, scraping sides of bowl occasionally. Use a rubber spatula to stir in apples and toasted nuts; mix until well blended.

Pour into prepared pan and bake 30 minutes or until pick inserted in center comes out clean. Cool on rack 20 minutes. Invert on a plate and remove pan. Turn cake right-side up on rack to cool completely, about 30 minutes. Place on serving plate and if desired, sprinkle with confectioners' sugar.   Store covered. Refrigerate after 2 days. Can be frozen up to 3 months.

SPICY APPLE
UPSIDE-DOWN CAKE

ROME OR GRANNY SMITH APPLES ARE PERFECT TO USE IN THIS CAKE
Prep time: 15 min   Bake time: 30 min
Serves: 8   Serving size: 1 Slice, 1/8 Portion
Exchanges: 1 Starch, 1/2 Fruit and 3 Fat (1 Carbohydrate Choice)
Analysis per serving: 212 Calories, 22 g Carbohydrate, 4 g Protein,
12 g Fat, 0 mg Cholesterol, 107 mg Sodium, 1 g Fiber

2	Tbs olive or canola oil
2	Tbs brown sugar
1	Tbs lemon juice
1	large baking apple, washed, cored & thinly sliced
1/2	cup whole-wheat flour
1/2	cup all-purpose flour
1/4	tsp salt
1/2	tsp cinnamon
1/8	tsp nutmeg
1/8	tsp cloves
1/2	cup egg substitute
1/3	cup olive or canola oil
1/3	cup skim milk
1/4	cup sugar
1	tsp butter extract
1/2	tsp vanilla extract

Preheat oven 350°F. Have an 8-inch round cake pan ready.

Measure 2 Tbs oil, brown sugar and lemon juice into pan and use a rubber spatula to mix well; spread evenly over bottom of pan. Bake 1 minute. Stir again and arrange apple slices, spoke fashion, over brown sugar mixture in pan. Press any additional apple slices onto sides of pan. Set aside.

In medium bowl, use rubber spatula to combine flours, salt and spices; add egg substitute, oil, milk, sugar and extracts. Use electric mixer at medium speed to beat mixture for 2 minutes, scraping bowl occasionally.

Spread batter over apple slices. Bake 30 to 35 minutes or until pick inserted in center comes out clean. Cool on rack 10 minutes. Use a knife to loosen cake and invert onto rack. Cool completely, at least 30 minutes before serving. Store covered. Can be frozen up to 3 months.

DATE NUT APPLE CAKE

A MOIST, CHEWY CAKE
Prep time: 15 min   Bake time: 55 min
Serves: 16   Serving size: 1 Slice, 1/16 Portion
Exchanges: 1 Starch, 1/2 Fruit and 2 Fat (1 Carbohydrate Choice)
Analysis per serving: 186 Calories, 22 g Carbohydrate, 3 g Protein,
10 g Fat, 26 mg Cholesterol, 102 mg Sodium, 2 g Fiber

1/2	cup chopped walnuts
1	cup all-purpose flour
3/4	cup whole-wheat flour
1	tsp baking powder
1	tsp baking soda
1	tsp cinnamon
1/2	tsp cloves
2	tsp cocoa
4	cups peeled, chopped tart apples (3 or 4 medium)
1/2	cup chopped dates
1/2	cup olive or canola oil
1/4	cup sugar
2	large eggs or 1/2 cup egg substitute
1/2	cup cooled coffee (or dissolve 1 tsp instant coffee in 1/2 cup boiling water; cool)

Preheat oven 350°F. Place nuts on baking sheet; bake 3 to 5 minutes or until toasted; set aside. Spray a 10-inch tube or bundt pan with cooking spray.

In small bowl, combine flours, baking powder, baking soda, spices and cocoa; set aside.

In medium bowl, combine apples, toasted nuts, dates and 1/2 cup of the flour mixture; toss together until fruit pieces are well coated; set aside.

In large bowl, with electric mixer at medium speed, combine oil, sugar and eggs until blended; scrape bowl. With beater at low speed, add flour mixture alternately with coffee, beginning and ending with flour mixture, until batter is smooth. Scrape bowl after each addition. Stir in fruit mixture and mix well. Spoon into prepared pan; smooth top.

Bake 55 to 60 minutes or until browned and pick inserted in center comes out clean. Cool on rack 20 minutes; remove from pan; cool completely on rack for about 1 hour. Store in refrigerator after 2 days. Can be frozen up to 3 months.

GRAND FINALE APPLE CAKE

A QUICK AND EASY CAKE WITH A SURPRISE INGREDIENT
Prep time: 20 min   Bake time: 75 min
Serves: 16   Serving size: 1 Slice, 1/16 Portion
Exchanges: 1 Starch, 1 Fruit and 2 Fat (2 Carbohydrate Choices)
Analysis per serving: 233 Calories, 33 g Carbohydrate, 4 g Protein,
10 g Fat, 26 mg Cholesterol, 146 mg Sodium, 3 Fiber

4	cups unpeeled, diced apples (3 or 4 medium)
1/2	cup sugar
1/2	cup chopped walnuts
1 1/2	cups whole-wheat flour
1 1/2	cups all-purpose flour
2	tsp baking soda
2	tsp cinnamon
1	tsp allspice
1/2	tsp nutmeg
1/2	tsp cloves
1/2	cup olive or canola oil
1/2	cup unsweetened applesauce
2	large eggs, beaten or 1/2 cup egg substitute
1	Tbs Worcestershire sauce
1/2	cup raisins

In medium bowl, combine chopped apples with sugar; set aside for 15 minutes.

Preheat oven to 325°F. Place nuts on baking sheet; bake 3 to 5 minutes or until toasted; set aside. Spray a 10-inch tube pan with cooking spray.

In large bowl, sift all dry ingredients. If grains remain in sifter, just add to dry ingredients. Use a rubber spatula to stir in oil, applesauce, eggs and Worcestershire sauce; blend thoroughly. Stir in apple mixture, raisins and toasted nuts; mix well, scraping sides of bowl.

Pour into prepared pan and bake 1 hour 15 minutes or until cake is browned and pick inserted in center comes out clean. Cool in pan on rack for 20 minutes. Use a knife to loosen cake and remove from pan; cool completely, about 1 hour, on rack. Refrigerate after 2 days.

BLUEBERRY BUNDT CAKE

A BURST OF BLUEBERRIES IN EVERY BITE
Prep time: 15 min　　　　　　　Bake time: 1 hr
Serves: 16　　　　　　　　　　Serving size: 1 Slice, 1/16 Portion
Exchanges: 1 Starch, 1/2 Fruit and 1 1/2 Fat (2 Carbohydrate Choices)
Analysis per serving: 177 Calories, 24 g Carbohydrate, 4 g Protein,
8 g Fat, 26 mg Cholesterol, 156 mg Sodium, 2 g Fiber

1	cup whole-wheat flour
1 1/4	cup all-purpose flour
2 1/2	tsp baking powder
1	tsp baking soda
1/4	tsp salt
1/2	tsp nutmeg
4	large egg whites, at room temperature
1/4	tsp cream of tartar
1/2	cup sugar, divided
2	large egg yolks, at room temperature
1/2	cup olive or canola oil
1/2	cup buttermilk
1/2	cup orange juice
2	cups (1 pint) fresh or frozen blueberries, washed & drained
1	tsp dried lemon peel or grated fresh lemon peel

Preheat oven to 350°F. Spray a 10-inch bundt or tube pan with cooking spray.

Sift flours, baking powder, baking soda and nutmeg into a small bowl. If grains remain in sifter, just add to sifted flour mixture; set aside.

In a medium bowl, with electric mixer at high speed, beat egg whites until frothy. Beat in cream of tartar at high speed until soft peaks form. Gradually beat in 1/4 cup sugar at high speed, scraping bowl occasionally, until peaks are stiff when batter is lifted with rubber spatula; set aside.

In a large bowl, using same beaters at medium speed, beat yolks and remaining 1/4 cup sugar, 1 to 2 minutes, or until thick and lemon-colored. Scrape bowl and beat in oil, buttermilk and orange juice at medium speed. Reserve 1/4 flour mixture; set aside. With beater at low speed, gradually beat in remaining sifted flour mixture; scrape sides of bowl. Combine blueberries and reserved flour mixture until berries are coated. Stir lemon peel and coated blueberries into batter. Use a rubber spatula to gently stir in stiffly beaten egg whites using an under and over motion until no white streaks remain.

Spoon batter into prepared pan. Bake 60 to 65 minutes or until lightly browned and pick inserted in center, comes out clean. Cool on rack for 20 minutes. Use a knife to loosen cake and remove from pan; cool on rack, about 1 hour. Store covered; refrigerate after 2 days. Can be frozen up to 3 months. Refer to pages 237-238 for freezing directions.

CARROT APPLESAUCE CAKE

A DELICIOUS WAY TO INCORPORATE BRAN INTO YOUR DIET
Prep time: 10 min   Bake time: 60 min
Serves: 16   Serving size: 1 Slice, 1/16 Portion
Exchanges: 1 Starch, 1/2 Fruit and 1 Fat (2 Carbohydrate Choices)
Analysis per serving: 154 Calories, 24 g Carbohydrate, 4 g Protein,
6 g Fat, 39 mg Cholesterol, 228 mg Sodium, 3 g Fiber

1	cup whole-wheat flour
1	cup all-purpose flour
1	Tbs baking soda
2	tsp cinnamon
1	tsp cloves
1	tsp nutmeg
1/2	cup wheat bran
3	large eggs or 3/4 cup egg substitute
1/2	cup sugar
1/3	cup olive or canola oil
1 1/2	tsp vanilla extract
1 2/3	cups unsweetened applesauce
3	cups (1-pound package) carrots or baby carrots, shredded

Preheat oven to 350°F. Spray a 10-inch tube or bundt pan with cooking spray.

In large bowl, sift flours, baking soda, spices and bran. If grains remain in sifter, just add to flour mixture; set aside.

In medium bowl, with electric mixer at medium speed, beat eggs, sugar, oil and vanilla until well mixed. Use a rubber spatula to stir in applesauce and shredded carrots until blended. Pour wet mixture into flour mixture and stir just to moisten; do not overmix.

Spoon batter into prepared pan and bake 60 to 65 minutes or until pick inserted in center comes out clean. Cool on rack 15 minutes. Use a knife to loosen cake, remove from pan and cool completely on rack about 1 hour. If desired, sprinkle with confectioners' sugar. Store covered. Refrigerate after 2 days.

PINEAPPLE CARROT CAKE

A TRADITIONAL CARROT CAKE
Prep time: 10 min   Bake time: 30 min
Serves: 16   Serving size: 1 Slice, 1/16 Portion
Exchanges: 2 Starch and 1 1/2 Fat (1 Carbohydrate Choice)
Analysis per serving: 171 Calories, 22 g Carbohydrate, 3 g Protein,
8 g Fat, 40 mg Cholesterol, 184 mg Sodium, 2 g Fiber

1/2	cup chopped nuts (optional)
3	large eggs or 3/4 cup egg substitute
1/2	cup olive or canola oil
1/2	cup sugar
1	8-ounce can juice-packed crushed pineapple
1	cup whole-wheat flour
1	cup all-purpose flour
1	tsp baking powder
2	tsp baking soda
1	tsp cinnamon
1/2	tsp nutmeg
1	tsp vanilla extract
3	cups (1-pound package) carrots or baby carrots, grated
1/2	cup raisins (optional)

Preheat oven to 350°F. If using nuts, place on baking sheet; bake 3 to 5 minutes until toasted; set aside. Spray a 13x9x2-inch baking pan with cooking spray.

In a large bowl, use electric mixer at medium speed to beat eggs until frothy. Beat in oil and sugar at medium speed until well blended; scrape sides of bowl. Add crushed pineapple with juice, flours, baking powder, baking soda, spices and vanilla and beat at low speed until well blended. Use a rubber spatula to stir in carrots and nuts and raisins, if using.

Spread batter into prepared pan and bake 30 to 35 minutes or until wooden pick inserted in center comes out clean. Cool completely, about 1 hour, on wire rack. Run a knife around sides of cake to loosen from pan. Invert onto rack and place right side up on serving plate. Sprinkle with confectioners' sugar or frost with LIGHT CREAM CHEESE FROSTING (page 78)

SPICY PUMPKIN CAKE

THIS CAKE HAS A HIGHER SUGAR CONTENT THAN OTHERS IN THIS BOOK
Prep time: 10 min   Bake time: 60 min
Serves: 16   Serving size: 1 Slice, 1/16 Portion
Exchanges: 2 Starch and 2 Fat (2 Carbohydrate Choices)
Analysis per serrving: 234 Calories, 35 g Carbohydrate, 6 g Protein,
9 g Fat, 40 mg Cholesterol, 130 mg Sodium, 3 g Fiber

1 1/2	cups whole-wheat flour
1 1/2	cups all-purpose flour
1	Tbs baking powder
1/2	tsp baking soda
1	tsp cinnamon
2	tsp pumpkin pie spice
3	large eggs or 3/4 cup egg substitute
1/2	cup sugar
1/2	cup packed brown sugar
1/2	cup vegetable oil
3/4	cup skim milk
1	16-ounce can of canned pumpkin (NOT pie filling)
1 1/2	cups old-fashioned oats

Preheat oven to 350°F. Spray a 10-inch tube pan or bundt pan with cooking spray.

In medium bowl, stir together flours, baking powder, baking soda and spices. If grains remain in sifter, add to dry ingredients; set aside.

In large bowl, with electric mixer at medium speed, beat eggs until frothy; add sugars and beat at medium speed until thick. Scrape sides of bowl and add oil, milk and pumpkin; beat at medium speed until well blended, scraping bowl occasionally. At low speed, mix in flour mixture until well blended. Use a rubber spatula to stir in dry oatmeal until all ingredients are well mixed.

Pour into prepared pan and bake 60 to 65 minutes or until pick inserted in center comes out clean. Place on rack and cool about 20 minutes. Use a knife to carefully loosen cake from pan and turn out onto rack to cool completely, about 1 hour. If desired, sprinkle with confectioners' sugar before serving. Store covered. Refrigerate after 2 days.

DELIGHTFUL STRAWBERRY SHORTCAKE

A DIFFERENT VERSION OF STRAWBERRY SHORTCAKE
Prep time: 5 min   Bake time: 20 min
Serves: 12   Serving size: 1 Slice, 1/12 Portion
Exchanges: 1 Starch and 1/2 Fruit (2 Carbohydrate Choices)
Analysis per serving: 128 Calories, 24 g Carbohydrate, 4 g Protein,
1 g Fat, 54 mg Cholesterol, 86 Sodium, 1 g Fiber (with cake)

1	cup **YOGURT CHEESE (page 83)**
1	tsp vanilla extract
1	tsp sugar
1/2	cup orange juice
1/4	cup red wine
1/4	cup sugar
1	Tbs plus 1 tsp cornstarch
1	tsp dried orange peel or grated fresh orange peel
1	cup sliced fresh strawberries
1	FEATHERLIGHT SPONGE CAKE (page 51)
1	cup fresh strawberry halves

In a small bowl, combine YOGURT CHEESE with vanilla and sugar.
Refrigerate, covered, until ready to use.

In a 4-cup measuring cup, combine orange juice, wine, sugar, cornstarch
and peel. Microwave on High for 3 minutes or until mixture boils; stir;
cover and chill 1 hour.

Up to an hour before serving, place 1 layer of sponge cake on plate. Stir
orange juice mixture; spread half of juice mixture over cake layer and
arrange sliced strawberries over juice mixture. Top with remaining cake
layer; spoon remaining orange mixture evenly over cake. Arrange
strawberry halves on top of cake; top with yogurt mixture. If desired,
garnish with a whole strawberry.

CREAM PUFFS

PUFFS MADE WITH BREAD FLOUR WILL BE LARGER AND CRISPIER
Prep time: 15 min   Bake time: 25 min
Servings: 8   Serving size: 1 Puff
Exchanges: 1/2 Starch and 1 Fat (1 Carbohydrate Choice)
Analysis per serving: 90 Calories, 6 g Carbohydrate, 2 g Protein,
6 g Fat, 53 mg Cholesterol, 89 mg Sodium, 0 g Fiber

1/2	**cup all-purpose flour or bread flour**
1/4	**tsp salt**
1/2	**cup water**
3	**Tbs olive or canola oil**
2	**large eggs**

Preheat oven 450°F. Spray baking sheet with cooking spray. Sift flour and salt into a small bowl; set aside.

In medium saucepan, combine water and oil over high heat. Bring to a boil. With wooden spoon, beat in flour and salt all at once and stir vigorously until mixture leaves sides of pan and forms a ball, about 1 minute.

Remove pot from heat and beat in eggs, one at a time, using a wooden spoon, whisk or a hand held electric beater, until mixture is smooth and shiny. Spoon onto cookie sheet in 8 mounds, leaving about 2 inches between them for spreading.

Bake 10 minutes. Reduce heat to 400°F and continue baking 15 to 20 minutes or until pastry is puffed and golden browned. Cool on rack. Just before serving: cut a slice horizontally from top of each puff; remove any soft dough from inside each puff. Spoon filling into each puff and replace top. Serve immediately.

❖ Try filling with chilled FABULOUS CHOCOLATE PUDDING (page 188) or SIMPLE VANILLA PUDDING (page 200) Puffs can be baked up to 2 days before filling. Store in a covered container. Slice and fill puffs just before serving as directed.

PETITE CREAMS PUFFS

HEAVENLY LITTLE BITES
Prep time: 15 min   Bake time: 20 min
Servings: 16   Serving size: 2 Puffs
Exchanges: 1/2 Starch and 1 Fat (1 Carbohydrate Choice)
Analysis per serving: 90 Calories, 6 g Carbohydrate, 2 g Protein,
6 g Fat, 53 mg Cholesterol, 89 mg Sodium, 0 g Fiber

Prepare puffs as directed in previous CREAM PUFFS recipe.

Drop cream puff mixture by rounded teaspoonfuls onto prepared baking sheet. Bake at 450°F for 5 minutes.

Reduce heat to 400°F and bake 10 to 15 minutes more or until puffed and golden brown.

Cool on rack and fill as desired just before serving.

❖ Puffs can be baked up to 2 days before filling. Store in a covered container. Slice and fill puffs just before serving as directed.

ORANGE ZUCCHINI CAKE

THIS RECIPE WORKS WELL BAKED AS A LOAF, BUNDT OR LAYER CAKE
Prep time: 15 min   Bake time: 30 min
Servings: 16   Serving size: 1 Slice, 1/16 Portion
Exchanges: 1 Starch, 1 Vegetable and 1 Fat (1 Carbohydrate Choice)
Analysis per serving: 163 Calories, 20 g Carbohydrate, 4 g Protein,
8 g Fat, 40 mg Cholesterol, 132 mg Sodium, 2 g Fiber

1/2	cup chopped nuts (optional)
1	cup whole-wheat flour
1	cup all-purpose flour
1/2	cup old-fashioned oats
2	tsp baking powder
1	tsp baking soda
2	tsp cinnamon
1/2	tsp cloves
1	tsp dried orange peel or grated fresh orange peel
3	large eggs or 3/4 cup egg substitute
1/2	cup olive or canola oil
1/4	cup brown sugar
1/4	cup sugar
1/2	cup unsweetened orange juice
1	tsp almond extract
2	cups zucchini, shredded (1 medium)

Preheat oven 350°F. If using nuts, place on baking sheet; bake 3 to 5 minutes or until toasted; set aside. Spray one of the following with cooking spray:

Pan Size	Bake
1 10-cup tube or bundt pan	55 to 60 min
1 13x9x2-inch pan	35 to 40 min
3 5x2-inch small loaf pans	40 to 45 min
2 8x4x2-inch loaf pans	40 to 45 min
2 8- or 9-inch square baking pans	30 to 35 min

In large bowl, use a rubber spatula to mix flours, baking powder, baking soda, spices and peel; set aside.

In another large bowl, use a whisk to beat eggs. Whisk in oil, sugars, juice, extract and zucchini. Add wet ingredients and toasted nuts (if using) to flour mixture, stirring just to moisten.

Pour into prepared pan(s) and bake until pick inserted in center comes out clean.   Cool in pan on rack for 10 minutes. Loosen cake from pan and invert onto rack to cool completely. Store covered. Refrigerate after 2 days or freeze up to 3 months.

COCOA ZUCCHINI CAKE

A SMALL AMOUNT OF COCOA GIVES THIS CAKE A DISTINCTIVE FLAVOR
Prep time: 15 min   Bake time: 45-60 min.
Serves: 16   Serving size: 1 Slice, 1/16 Portion
Exchanges: 1 1/2 Starch and 1/2 Fat (2 Carbohydrate Choices)
Analysis per serving: 138 Calories, 23 g Carbohydrate, 4 g Protein,
4 g Fat, 13 mg Cholesterol, 157 mg Sodium, 2 g Fiber

1/2	cup sugar
1/4	cup olive or canola oil
1/4	cup unsweetened applesauce
1/2	cup skim milk
1	tsp vanilla extract
1	large egg
2	large egg whites
1	cup whole-wheat flour
1 1/2	cups all-purpose flour
1/4	cup cocoa
1	tsp baking soda
1/2	tsp cinnamon
1/2	tsp salt
2	cups unpeeled zucchini, shredded (1 medium)

Preheat oven to 350°F. Spray a 10-inch bundt pan or a 13x9x2-inch pan with cooking spray.

In large bowl, use electric mixer at medium speed to beat sugar, oil, applesauce, milk, vanilla, egg and egg whites until well blended; scrape sides of bowl.

Sift flours, cocoa, baking soda, cinnamon and salt into a small bowl or onto wax paper. If grains remain in sifter, add to dry ingredients. With mixer at low speed, beat in flour mixture and shredded zucchini alternately with egg mixture, beginning and ending with flour mixture. Mix well, scraping bowl occasionally.

Pour into either prepared pan.   Bake 60 minutes for bundt pan or 45 minutes for 13x9x2-inch pan or until pick inserted in center comes out clean. Cool on rack for 10 or 15 minutes; loosen cake and remove from cake pan and cool completely on rack, about 1 hour. Store covered. Refrigerate covered after 2 days. Delicious sliced and toasted.

SPEEDY CHOCOLATE CAKE

APPLESAUCE TAKES THE PLACE OF OIL ADDING FLAVOR AND TEXTURE
Prep time: 5 min   Bake time: 20 min
Serves: 9   Serving size: 1 Slice, 1/9 Portion
Exchanges: 1 Starch and 1 Fat (1 Carbohydrate Choice)
Analysis per serving: 115 Calories, 19 g Carbohydrate, 4 g Protein,
3 g Fat, 0 mg Cholesterol, 243 mg Sodium, 2 g Fiber

2	squares (1 ounce each) unsweetened baking chocolate
1/4	cup whole-wheat flour
1/2	cup all-purpose flour
1/3	cup sugar
2	tsp baking powder
1	tsp baking soda
3/4	tsp cinnamon
1/2	cup unsweetened applesauce
1/2	cup skim milk
1/2	cup egg substitute
1	tsp vanilla extract

Place chocolate squares in custard cup. Microwave on High 1 minute, stir; microwave on High for another minute or so until melted; set aside.

Preheat oven to 375°F. Spray a 9-inch square pan with cooking spray.

In large bowl, mix flours, sugar, baking powder, baking soda and cinnamon together until well blended. Add applesauce, milk, egg substitute, vanilla and melted chocolate; beat rapidly with a wooden spoon or 1 minute with electric mixer at medium speed until smooth. Scrape bowl, mix and pour into prepared pan.

Bake 20 to 25 minutes or until pick inserted in center comes out clean and sides pull away from pan. Cool 10 minutes on rack. Cut into squares to serve warm or at room temperature. If desired, sprinkle with confectioners' sugar. Delicious served with fresh fruit and WHIPPED TOPPING (page 79).

CHOCOLATE CLOUD CAKE

EGG WHITES MAKE THIS NONFAT CHOCOLATE CAKE LIGHT AND AIRY
Prep time: 15 min   Bake time: 20 min
Serves: 8   Serving size: 1 Slice, 1/8 Portion
Exchanges: 1 Fruit (1 Carbohydrate Choice)
Analysis per serving: 63 Calories, 14 g Carbohydrate, 3 g Protein,
0 g Fat, 0 mg Cholesterol, 204 mg Sodium, 0 g Fiber

1/3	cup cocoa
1/3	cup water
1/2	tsp vanilla extract
1/4	cup all-purpose flour
2	tsp baking powder
4	large egg whites, at room temperature
1/4	tsp salt
1/3	cup sugar
	Confectioners' sugar

Preheat oven to 350°F. Have an 8-inch round cake pan ready. Place cake pan on a piece of wax paper. Trace pan and cut out wax paper to fit on bottom of pan; set aside.

In 1-cup glass measuring cup, use a small whisk to mix cocoa and water. Microwave on High 1 minute, stir, microwave 1 more minute or until thick and smooth. Stir in vanilla; cool. In separate small bowl, blend flour and baking powder together. Set aside.

In large bowl, with electric mixer at high speed, beat egg whites and salt until foamy. Gradually beat in sugar at high speed until soft peaks form when batter is lifted with rubber spatula. Immediately add cocoa mixture and beat just until blended; scrape sides of bowl. Use a rubber spatula to fold in flour mixture just until blended. Do not over mix.

Pour into prepared pan and smooth top with rubber spatula. Bake 20 to 25 minutes or until top cracks and looks dry and pick inserted in center comes out dry. Place cake, still in pan, upside down on wire rack on top of piece of wax paper that has been spray with cooking spray; cool 20 minutes. Turn right side up; remove wax paper from top of cake and run knife around sides of pan to loosen.   Carefully turn out onto rack to cool; remove wax paper; turn right side up.   Cool completely, about 30 minutes.

To serve, place doily over cake and sprinkle with confectioners' sugar. Carefully remove doily.

Diabetic Goodie Book

CHOCOLATE UPSIDE CAKE

AN UPSIDE DOWN CAKE WITH A RICH BROWNIE TASTE
Prep time: 15 min   Bake time: 40 min
Serves: 9   Serving size: 1 Slice, 1/9 Portion
Exchanges: 1 1/2 Starch and 2 Fat (1 Carbohydrate Choice)
Analysis per serving: 177 Calories, 21 g Carbohyrate, 4 g Protein,
10 g Fat, 24 mg Cholesterol, 184 mg Sodium, 2 g Fiber

2	squares (1 ounce each) unsweetened baking chocolate
2	Tbs olive or canola oil
1	Tbs brown sugar
1/3	cup chopped walnuts
2	Tbs sugar
1/4	cup unsweetened applesauce
1/2	cup mashed ripe banana (1 medium)
1	large egg or 1/4 cup egg substitute
1	cup cake flour
2	tsp baking powder
1/4	tsp salt
3/4	cup buttermilk

Place chocolate squares in custard cup. Microwave on High for 1
minutes; stir. Microwave another minute or until melted; stir. Set aside.

Preheat oven to 350°F. Spray 8-inch square pan with cooking spray and
add oil and brown sugar. Use a rubber spatula to mix and spread mixture
evenly in bottom of pan. Place in oven for 2 minutes to melt brown sugar
mixture. Add nuts and stir until nuts are coated; spread evenly in pan. Set
aside.

In medium bowl, with electric mixer at medium speed, beat sugar,
applesauce, banana, egg and melted chocolate, scraping bowl
occasionally, until well blended, about 2 minutes.

Sift cake flour, baking powder and salt onto waxed paper or into a small
bowl. If grains remain in sifter, add to dry ingredients. With mixer at
medium speed, add flour mixture and buttermilk alternately to batter,
beginning and ending with flour mixture. Mix and scrape bowl until well
blended.

Pour into pan and bake 40 minutes or until pick inserted in center comes
out clean. Cool on rack 5 minutes. Use a knife to loosen edges of cake
from pan; invert on plate, remove pan and cool on plate on rack about 30
minutes.

ITALIAN CHOCOLATE ROLL

A SPECTACULAR DESSERT!
Prep time: 20 min   Bake time: 15 min   Chill time: 4 hrs
Serves: 10   Serving size: 1 Slice, 1/10 Portion
Exchanges: 1 Low-fat milk (1 Carbohydrate Choice)
Analysis per serving: 110 Calories, 13 g Carbohydate, 10 g Protein,
3 g Fat, 57 mg Cholesterol, 110 mg Sodium, 0 g Fiber

Cake

1/4	cup cocoa
2	Tbs all-purpose flour
1/8	tsp salt
4	large eggs, separated and at room temperature
1/2	tsp cream of tartar
1/3	cup confectioners' sugar, sifted
1	tsp vanilla extract
	Confectioners' sugar

Preheat oven to 325°F. Spray a 15x10x1-inch jelly roll pan with cooking spray. Line with waxed paper or parchment paper and spray again; set aside.

Sift cocoa, flour and salt into a small bowl; set aside.

In medium bowl, with electric mixer at high speed, beat egg whites until frothy; beat in cream of tartar at high speed and beat until stiff peaks form when batter is lifted with rubber spatula.

With same beaters, in another medium bowl, beat yolks at medium speed until thick and lemon colored, 2 to 3 minutes. Gradually beat in sifted confectioners' sugar and vanilla at medium speed; scrape bowl. Use a rubber spatula to stir in cocoa mixture. Using the rubber spatula, gently fold beaten whites, half at a time, into yolk mixture until no white streaks remain.

Spoon into prepared pan and smooth with rubber spatula. Bake 12 to 15 minutes or until center springs back when lightly pressed. Meanwhile, prepare filling.

Filling

2	cups nonfat ricotta cheese
1	Tbs finely chopped blanched almonds, toasted
2	Tbs dark rum
3	Tbs sugar
2	tsp dried orange peel or grated fresh orange peel
1	Tbs mini chocolate chips
1/2	tsp vanilla extract

In medium bowl, with electric mixer at low speed, beat ricotta until smooth. Use a rubber spatula to stir in toasted nuts, rum, sugar, peel, chips and vanilla until well blended.

Lay a clean dishtowel on counter and sprinkle with sifted confectioners' sugar.

Remove cake from oven and loosen edges with knife. Place cake side down on prepared towel; lift off baking pan and peel off paper. Starting at short end, roll up cake and towel. Place seam side down on rack to cool about 15 minutes. Unroll cake and spread filling to within 1/2-inch of edges. Using towel as a guide, reroll cake with filling. Place seam side down on serving plate; cover. Refrigerate at least one hour or up to 4 hours before serving. Sprinkle cake with sifted confectioners' sugar before serving.

STRAWBERRY PINEAPPLE ROLL

YOU'LL GET RAVE REVIEWS WHEN YOU SERVE THIS CAKE ROLL
Prep time: 20 min   Bake time: 30 min
Serves: 12   Serving size: 1 Slice, 1/12 Portion
Exchanges: 1 Starch and 1 Skim milk (2 Carbohydrate Choices)
Analysis per serving: 146 Calories, 23 g Carbohydrate, 9 g Protein,
2 g Fat, 70 mg Cholesterol, 152 mg Sodium, 1 g Fiber

Cake

1/2	cup all-purpose flour
1/4	cup whole-wheat flour
1	tsp baking powder
1/4	tsp salt
4	large eggs
1/2	cup sugar
2	Tbs water
1	tsp vanilla extract

Confectioners' sugar

Preheat oven to 350°F. Spray a 15x10x1-inch jelly roll pan with cooking spray, line with waxed paper or parchment paper and spray again.

In a small bowl, combine flours, baking powder and salt; set aside. In large bowl, using electric mixer at medium speed, beat eggs until frothy; gradually beat in sugar until thick and pale. Scrape bowl; beat in water and vanilla at low speed. Use rubber spatula to stir in reserved dry ingredients until well blended.

Pour batter into prepared pan; spread evenly with rubber spatula. Bake 15 to 20 minutes or until cake pulls away from sides of pan and center springs back when pressed.

Meanwhile, dust a clean dish towel with sifted confectioners' sugar and prepare filling.

Filling

1	8-ounce can juice-packed crushed pineapple, drained, juice reserved
2	cups nonfat ricotta cheese
2	Tbs sugar
2	Tbs nonfat plain yogurt
1	tsp rum extract
2	cups (1 pint) fresh strawberries, washed & drained

Drain pineapple, reserving juice; set pineapple and juice aside. In medium bowl, with electric mixer at low speed, beat ricotta until smooth. Beat in 3 Tbs of reserved pineapple juice, sugar, yogurt and rum extract until well blended, scrape bowl. Use a rubber spatula to stir in reserved crushed pineapple.

Loosen cake around edges with a knife and place cake side down on prepared towel; remove pan and gently peel off paper. Starting from one long side, roll cake and towel together; cool on rack about 15 minutes. Unroll cooled cake. Reserve 1 cup of filling. Spread remainder on cake to within 1/2-inch of edges. Reserve 4 whole berries; hull and slice remainder. Spoon sliced berries evenly over filling. Roll up cake and filling from same long side using towel as a guide; place seam side down on a large serving plate. Prepare, cover and refrigerate at least 1 hour or up to 4 hours before serving. Sprinkle with confectioners' sugar; garnish with reserved berries.

To serve, cut in 12 slices and pass reserved filling to spoon on each serving.

PUMPKIN CHEESE ROLL

UNIQUE CAKE BRIMMING WITH SPICY FLAVOR
Prep time: 20 min   Bake time: 20 min
Serves: 10   Serving size: 1 Slice, 1/10 Portion
Exchanges: 1 Starch, 1 Skim milk and 1 Fat (2 Carbohydrate Choices)
Analysis per serving: 213 Calories, 25 g Carbohydrate, 9 g Protein,
9 g Fat, 63 mg Cholesterol, 236 mg Sodium, 1 g Fiber

Cake

1/2	cup all-purpose flour
1/4	cup whole-wheat flour
1	tsp baking powder
2	tsp cinnamon
1	tsp ginger
1/2	tsp nutmeg
1/4	tsp salt
3	large eggs, slightly beaten
1/2	cup sugar
2/3	cup canned or cooked pumpkin (NOT pie filling)
1	tsp lemon juice
1	cup finely chopped nuts
	Confectioners' sugar

Preheat oven to 375°F. Spray a 15x10x1-inch jelly roll pan with cooking spray. Line with waxed paper or parchment paper and spray again.

Sift flours, baking powder, spices and salt into a small bowl. If grains remain in sifter, stir into dry ingredients.

In large bowl, with electric beater at medium speed, beat eggs and sugar until thick, about 3 minutes. Beat in pumpkin and lemon juice at medium speed; scrape sides of bowl. Using a rubber spatula, stir in dry ingredients all at once until well blended.

Pour into prepared pan, spread evenly with rubber spatula. Sprinkle nuts evenly. Bake 12 to 15 minutes or until top springs back when lightly touched.

Meanwhile, sprinkle a clean dishtowel with sifted confectioners' sugar. Prepare filling.

Filling

1	**8-ounce package nonfat cream cheese, softened**
1/4	**cup confectioners' sugar**
1	**tsp vanilla extract**
1/3	**cup nonfat ricotta cheese**
2	**tsp butter extract**

In small bowl, with electric mixer at medium speed, beat cream cheese until smooth. Scrape bowl and beat in confectioners' sugar, vanilla, ricotta cheese and butter extract until light and fluffy, about 30 seconds, scraping bowl occasionally.

Remove cake from oven and loosen cake around edges with a knife. Place cake top down on prepared towel, lift off pan and gently peel off waxed paper. Beginning at short end, roll cake and towel together. Set seam side down on a rack to cool, about 15 minutes. Unroll cake and spread with filling to within 1/2-inch of edges. Reroll cake, set seam side down on plate. Cover and refrigerate at least 1 hour or up to 4 hours before serving. Nuts will be on outside of cake.

YUMMY CHOCOLATE CUPCAKES

> **WONDERFUL TO MAKE WITH CHILDREN, SO QUICK & SIMPLE!**
> Prep time: 5 min   Bake time: 15 min
> Makes: 12 Cupcakes   Serving size: 1 Cupcake
> Exchanges: 1 1/2 Starch and 1 Fat (2 Carbohydrate Choices)
> Analysis per serving: 155 Calories, 26 g Carbohydrate, 2 g Protein,
> 5 g Fat, 0 mg Cholesterol, 141 mg Sodium, 3 g Fiber

3/4	**cup whole-wheat flour**
3/4	**cup all-purpose flour**
1/2	**cup sugar**
1/2	**cup cocoa**
1	**tsp baking soda**
1/4	**tsp salt**
3/4	**cup orange juice**
3	**Tbs olive or canola oil**
1	**Tbs white vinegar**
1	**tsp vanilla extract**
1/2	**cup water**
1/3	**cup mini chocolate chips**

Preheat oven to 375°F. Spray muffin pan with cooking spray or line with paper liners.

In a large bowl, combine flours, sugar, cocoa, baking soda and salt. Make a well in center and orange juice, oil, vinegar, vanilla and water. Stir just to moisten. Add chips and mix gently to combine.

Spoon into prepared pan and bake about 15 minutes or until pick inserted in center comes out clean. Immediately remove cupcakes from pan and cook completely on rack. Makes 12 regular-sized cupcakes.

❖ May also be baked in mini-muffins pans which have been sprayed with cooking spray or lined with miniature paper liners. Bake about 10 minutes or until pick inserted in center comes out clean. Makes about 3 1/2 dozen mini cupcakes.

HEALTHY HOLIDAY FRUITCAKE

SIMPLY DELICIOUS!
Prep time: 20 min   Bake time: 60 min
Makes: 2 Loaves   Serving size: 1 Slice, 1/20 Portion
Exchanges: 1 Starch, 1 Fruit and 2 Fat (1 Carbohydrate Choice)
Analysis per serving: 169 Calories, 22 g Carbohydrate, 3 g Protein,
9 g Fat, 25 mg Cholesterol, 64 mg Sodium, 2 g Fiber

1/3	cup unsalted light butter, softened
2	Tbs brown sugar
2	large eggs or 1/2 cup egg substitute
2	Tbs honey
1/4	cup whole-wheat flour
1/4	cup all-purpose flour
1/4	tsp salt
1/2	tsp baking powder
1/2	tsp cinnamon
1/8	tsp ground allspice
1/8	tsp nutmeg
2	Tbs evaporated skim milk
1/2	cup raisins
1	cup chopped dates
1	cup dried apricots, finely chopped
2	cups pecan halves

Preheat oven 300°F. Spray two 7 3/4 X 3 5/8 X 2 1/4-inch loaf pans with cooking spray. Line with aluminum foil and spray again; set aside.

In a large bowl, use an electric mixer at medium speed to cream butter, sugar, eggs and honey.

In a small bowl, combine flours, salt and spices. Add to creamed mixture alternately with skimmed evaporated milk, beginning and ending with flour mixture. Stir in raisins, dates, apricots and nuts until well blended and fruit and nuts are well coated with batter.

Spoon into prepared pans and spread evenly. Place filled pans on middle rack of oven. Place a shallow pan of hot water on lowest rack.Bake for 60 to 65 minutes or until pick inserted in center, comes out clean.

Place on rack to cool about 10 minutes. Remove fruitcakes with foil to rack to cool completely. Remove foil and store in airtight container or plastic storage bag in refrigerator. Use a serrated knife to slice.

LIGHT CREAM CHEESE FROSTING

TEMPTING FAT-FREE FROSTING
Prep time: 15 min   Cook time: 1 min
Makes: 1 1/2 Cups   Serving size: 1 Tbs, 1/24 Portion
Exchanges: Free; 2 Tbs = 1/2 Starch
Analysis per serving: 18 Calories, 3 g Carbohydrate, 1 g Protein,
0 g Fat, 1 mg Cholesterol, 50 mg Sodium, 0 g Fiber

1/4	cup sugar
2	Tbs orange juice
Pasteurized dried egg white	for 1 egg white
Water	(see page 13)
1	8-ounce package nonfat cream cheese, softened
1/2	tsp dried orange peel or grated fresh orange peel
1/2	tsp vanilla extract

In 1-cup glass measuring cup, microwave sugar and orange juice for 1 minute; stir.

In small bowl, using electric mixer at high speed, beat dried egg white powder and water until soft peaks form; gradually add sugar mixture in a thin stream. Continue beating at high speed until mixture is thick and glossy, about 4 minutes; scrape bowl occasionally.

In medium bowl, using same beaters at high speed, beat cream cheese, orange peel and vanilla until light and fluffy, about 5 minutes; scrape bowl occasionally. Add 1/3 of egg white mixture to cream cheese mixture, beating at low speed, just until blended. Using a rubber spatula, gently fold in remaining egg white mixture until it is completely blended into cream cheese mixture.

Frost cake and store covered in refrigerator.

WHIPPED TOPPING

IF TOPPING LOSES VOLUME AFTER CHILLING, REWHIP
Prep time: 5 min   Cook time: 0 min
Makes: 2 Cups   Serving size: 1/4 Cup, 1/8 Portion
Exchanges: 1/2 Skim milk
Analysis per serving: 42 Calories, 4 g Carbohydrate, 3 g Protein,
0 g Fat, 1 mg Cholesterol, 41 mg Sodium, 0 g Fiber

1/2	cup cold water
1	Tbs lemon juice
1	envelope unflavored gelatin
1/2	cup nonfat dry milk powder
2	Tbs sugar
1/4	tsp vanilla extract

Place a small bowl and beaters in refrigerator for at least one hour before preparing this recipe.

In a small chilled bowl, with electric mixer at medium speed, beat water, lemon juice and gelatin with chilled beaters until well blended. Gradually beat in dry milk at medium speed until moistened, scraping sides of bowl occasionally. Turn mixer to high speed and beat mixture until light and fluffy, scraping sides of bowl occasionally until soft peaks form when mixture is lifted with rubber spatula. Scrape sides of bowl and gradually beat in sugar and vanilla at high speed until stiff peaks form.

Serve at once. Store leftovers, covered, in refrigerator. Makes about 2 cups.

EASY FAT-FREE TOPPING

QUICK, EASY & FAT FREE!
Prep time: 5 min   Cook time: 0 min
Makes: 3 Cups   Serving size: 1/4 Cup, 1/12 Portion
Exchanges: 1/4 Skim milk
Analysis per serving: 26 Calories, 4 g Carbohydrate, 2 g Protein,
0 g Fat, 2 mg Cholesterol, 32 mg Sodium, 0 g Fiber

1	**12-ounce can evaporated skim milk**
1	**Tbs sugar**
1	**tsp vanilla extract**

One hour before preparing topping, place unopened can of evaporated skim milk in freezer. At same time, refrigerate small whipping bowl and beaters.

Shake can and pour cold milk into refrigerated bowl. Using electric mixer at high speed, beat cold evaporated milk with cold beaters until slightly stiff; gradually beat in sugar and vanilla at high speed, scraping bowl occasionally, until very stiff when mixture is lifted with a rubber spatula.

Serve immediately. Makes about 3 cups.

❖ If milk doesn't whip well, it needs to be colder. Put the bowl filled with milk and beaters back in the freezer for about 15 minutes and then try again.

TEMPTING
BLUEBERRY TOPPING

A FLAVORFUL TOPPING FOR CHEESECAKE, WAFFLES OR PANCAKES
Prep time: 10 min   Cook time: 0 min
Makes: 1 1/2 Cups   Serving size: 1 Tbs, 1/24 Portion
Exchanges: Free; 2 Tbs = 1/2 Starch
Analysis per serving: 18 Calories, 3 g Carbohydrate, 1 g Protein,
0 g Fat, 1 mg Cholesterol, 50 mg Sodium, 0 g Fiber

2	Tbs cornstarch
1/2	cup water, divided
1 1/4	cups fresh or frozen blueberries
2	Tbs honey
2	tsp lemon juice

In a 4-cup glass measuring cup, use a whisk or fork to mix cornstarch and 2 Tbs of water from the 1/2 cup of water until smooth. Use a wooden spoon to stir in remaining water, blueberries and honey until well mixed. Microwave on High for 2 minutes; stir. Microwave 2 to 6 minutes or until thickened and translucent, stirring every 2 minutes. Stir in lemon juice.

Cool before spreading on cake or cheesecake. Cool slightly before topping pancakes or waffles.   Store, covered, in refrigerator.

❖ Excellent topping for BLUEBERRY BUNDT CAKE (page 56), CREAMY RICOTTA CHEESECAKE (page 88) or KATHY'S CHEESECAKE (page 92).

Cheesecakes

Cheesecakes are a tempting treat. They represent decadence and luxury and a stylish, elegant close to a special meal. They are also a daring deviation from an ordinary birthday cake.

Here are 14 recipes that won't set you back on fat or calories. Nonfat ricotta cheese and nonfat cream cheese keep them creamy. Apples, peaches, kiwi, pineapple and pumpkin offer tempting variations.

Yogurt Cheese is a versatile ingredient in many kitchens. Besides making delicious cracker spreads, it is a terrific and easy part of several of these recipes. Here's how to make it.

YOGURT CHEESE
Place plain, nonfat yogurt into cheese cloth or a coffee filter. Place this in a strainer over a small bowl or cup. Allow it to drain for 2 to 24 hours, covered and refrigerated, until the cheese reaches a desired consistency.

Approximately half the yogurt will become cheese and half will become whey. Discard the whey.

Store Yogurt Cheese in a covered container in the refrigerator. Whey may continue releasing; just pour off and discard.

NO-BAKE SWIRL CHEESECAKE

NO NEED TO PUT THE OVEN ON TO MAKE THIS CREAMY CHEESECAKE
Prep time: 15 min   Chill time: 4 hrs
Serves: 8   Serving size: 1 Slice, 1/8 Portion
Exchanges: 2 Lean meat, 1/2 Skim milk and 1 Fruit (2 Carbohydrate Choices)
Analysis per serving: 204 Calories, 23 g Carbohydrate, 18 g Protein,
2 g Fat, 80 mg Cholesterol, 214 mg Sodium, 0 g Fiber

1/2	cup graham cracker crumbs
Pasteurized dried egg white for 3 egg whites	
Water	(see page 13)
4	Tbs sugar, divided
2	envelopes unflavored gelatin
3	large egg yolks
1 1/2	cups skim milk
3	cups nonfat ricotta cheese
3	Tbs lemon juice
2	tsp dried orange peel or grated fresh orange peel
1/2	tsp dried lemon peel or grated fresh lemon peel
1	tsp vanilla extract
1/4	cup nonfat dry milk powder
1/3	cup low-sugar raspberry jam

Have all ingredients at room temperature. Spray an 8-inch springform pan with cooking spray and wrap double layers of aluminum foil around outside of pan to prevent leakage. Sprinkle inside of prepared pan with crumbs. Refrigerate.

In large bowl, beat dried egg whites and water with electric beater at high speed until soft peaks form; gradually beat in 2 Tbs sugar until stiff peaks form when lifted with rubber spatula. Set aside.

In 4-cup glass measuring cup, mix remaining 2 Tbs sugar and gelatin. Add yolks and using same beaters, beat at medium speed until light and frothy; beat in milk. Microwave on Medium/High for 3 minutes. Stir, microwave on Medium/High for 6 minutes, stirring every 2 minutes, or until mixture forms a custard thick enough to coat a spoon.

Process ricotta in food processor or blender until smooth. Stir into custard along with lemon juice, peels, vanilla and dry milk until well blended. Using a rubber spatula, gently fold cheese mixture into beaten egg whites until no white streaks remain. Remove prepared pan from refrigerator and pour in ricotta mixture spreading mixture evenly.

In a 1-cup glass measuring cup, microwave jam on High 20 to 30 seconds until melted; stir. Drizzle melted raspberry jam over mixture and swirl with knife to marbleize. Cover carefully with plastic wrap so wrap does not touch cheesecake. Refrigerate at least 4 hours or overnight.

To serve, carefully loosen sides of cake with sharp knife. Remove sides of pan and leaving cake on pan bottom, place on serving plate. Cover and refrigerate leftovers.

NO-BAKE PEACHY RICOTTA CHEESECAKE

A TASTY NO-CRUST CHEESECAKE
Prep time: 20 min   Chill time: 4 hrs
Serves: 10   Serving size: 1 Slice, 1/10 Portion
Exchanges: 1 Skim milk, 1 Very lean meat and 1 Fruit (2 Carbohydrate Choices)
Analysis per serving: 173 Calories, 23 g Carbohydrate, 15 g Protein,
2 g Fat, 64 mg Cholesterol, 248 mg Sodium and 1 g Fiber

2	16-ounce cans juice-packed sliced peaches
Pasteurized dried egg white for 3 egg whites	
Water	(see page 13)
4	Tbs sugar, divided
2	envelopes unflavored gelatin
3	large egg yolks
1	tsp vanilla extract
1/4	tsp almond extract
3	cups nonfat ricotta cheese
1/2	cup nonfat dry milk powder
1	Tbs lemon juice
2	tsp dried orange peel or grated fresh orange peel
1/2	tsp dried lemon peel or grated fresh lemon peel

Have all ingredients at room temperature. Drain peaches; set drained peaches and juice aside. Spray a 9-inch springform pan with cooking spray.

In small bowl, beat dried egg whites and water with electric mixer at high speed until soft peaks form. Gradually beat in 2 Tbs sugar until stiff peaks form when lifted with rubber spatula; set aside.

In 4-cup glass measuring cup combine remaining 2 Tbs sugar and gelatin. With same beaters, add egg yolks and beat at medium speed until well blended, scraping sides occasionally; beat in vanilla and reserved peach juice. Microwave gelatin mixture on High for 3 minutes, stir and microwave another 2 minutes or until mixture comes to a boil; set aside to cool.

In food processor or blender, process ricotta and dry milk until smooth, scrape sides. With machine running, gradually drop in 1 cup of reserved peaches just until small pieces of peach are visible; scrape sides. In large bowl, combine peach mixture, gelatin mixture; lemon juice and dried peels; mix well. Use a rubber spatula to gently fold beaten egg whites into peach mixture until no white streaks remain. Pour mixture into prepared pan, spreading evenly.

Slice each peach slice into 2 thin slices and arrange slices on top of cheesecake in a circular manner. Cover with plastic wrap so wrap does not touch cake and refrigerate at least 4 hours or overnight.

To serve, use a sharp knife to loosen cake from pan. Remove sides of pan, leaving cake on pan bottom. Place on serving plate. Cover and refrigerate leftovers.

CREAMY RICOTTA CHEESECAKE

A DELICIOUS END TO AN ITALIAN MEAL!
Prep time: 10 min   Bake time: 50 min Chill time: 4 hrs
Serves: 10   Serving size: 1 Slice, 1/10 Portion
Exchanges: 1 Starch and 2 Very lean meat (1 Carbohydrate Choice)
Analysis per serving: 150 Calories, 15 g Carbohydrate, 15 Protein,
1 g Fat, 43 mg Cholesterol, 188 mg Sodium, 0 g Fiber

1/2	cup graham cracker crumbs
3 3/4	cups nonfat ricotta cheese
1/3	cup sugar
1	Tbs cornstarch
2	large eggs or 1/2 cup egg substitute
2	tsp vanilla extract
3	large egg whites
2	Tbs lemon juice
1	cup buttermilk
1	tsp dried lemon peel or grated fresh lemon peel

Preheat oven 375°F. Spray a 9-inch springform pan with cooking spray.
Sprinkle with graham cracker crumbs. Refrigerate while preparing filling.
Have 13x9x2-inch pan ready.

In food processor or with mixer, combine remaining ingredients. Process
until blended and smooth, scraping sides occasionally. Pour into prepared
pan and place in oven. Place 13x9x2-inch pan on shelf below cake and
fill with about 1-inch of hot water.   (This will prevent cheesecake from
cracking.)

Bake 50 to 60 minutes or until set. Shut off oven and leave oven door ajar
1-inch for 1 hour. Remove cheesecake from oven and cool on rack for 1
hour. Cover with plastic wrap and refrigerate at least 4 hours or overnight.
To serve, loosen sides of cake with sharp knife. Remove sides of pan
and leaving cake on pan bottom, place on serving plate.   If desired, serve
with sliced fresh fruit or a fruit topping of your choice. Refrigerate
leftovers covered.

CHOCOLATE CHEESECAKE

CHOCOLATE AND CHEESECAKE IN ONE FAST-FIXING DESSERT!
Prep time: 10 min   Bake time: 30 min Chill time: 3 hrs
Serves: 8   Serving size: 1 Slice, 1/8 Portion
Exchanges: 1 Starch, 1/2 Skim milk and 1 Fat (1 Carbohydrate Choice)
Analysis per serving: 176 Calories, 22 g Carbohydrate, 11 g Protein,
4 g Fat, 0 mg Cholesterol, 140 mg Sodium, 1 g Fiber

Crust

3/4	cup graham cracker crumbs
1/2	tsp cinnamon
2	Tbs sugar
2	Tbs olive or canola oil

Preheat oven 350°F. Spray 8-inch springform pan with cooking spray.
Fill a 13x9x2-inch pan half way with hot water. Place in oven on shelf
below where chocolate cheesecake will be placed.   This will prevent the
top of cheesecake from cracking.

In small bowl, combine all crust ingredients. Press onto bottom and
part-way up sides of pan. Set aside.

Filling

3	large egg whites
1/3	cup sugar
2	cups nonfat ricotta cheese
1/4	cup cocoa
1/3	cup YOGURT CHEESE (page 83)
1	tsp vanilla extract

In food processor or blender, combine egg whites, sugar, ricotta, cocoa,
yogurt cheese and vanilla; process, scraping sides occasionally, for 1
minute, until smooth and thick. Pour into crust.

Bake 30 to 35 minutes until filling is just set (center will jiggle slightly).
Turn off oven and leave cake in closed oven 5 minutes longer. Remove
from oven and cool about 1 hour on wire rack. Cover and refrigerate at
least 3 hours before serving.

BERRY CREAMY CHEESECAKE

EGGLESS CHEESECAKE WITH LUSCIOUS CREAMINESS
Prep time: 10 min   Bake time: 7 min Chill time: 3 hrs
Serves: 8   Serving size: 1 Slice, 1/8 Portion
Exchanges: 1 Starch, 1 Skim milk and 1 Fat (2 Carbohydrate Choices)
Analysis per serving: 220 Calories, 25 g Carbohydrate, 13 g Protein,
7 g Fat, 2 mg Cholesterol, 208 mg Sodium, 2 g Fiber

Crust

1	cup graham cracker crumbs
1	Tbs sugar
1/4	cup finely chopped pecans
2	Tbs olive or canola oil

Heat oven 350°F. Spray an 8-inch springform pan with cooking spray.

In small bowl, mix all ingredients. Press evenly over bottom and part-way up sides of pan. Bake 7 to 9 minutes or until lightly browned. Cool on wire rack before filling.

Filling

2	envelopes unflavored gelatin
2	cups buttermilk, divided
1/4	cup sugar
1	tsp dried lemon peel or grated fresh lemon peel
1	tsp strawberry extract (optional)
1	Tbs lemon juice
2	cups (16 ounces) nonfat cottage cheese
2	cups fresh strawberries, washed, drained & hulled, divided
1/2	cup fresh blueberries, washed & drained
1	kiwi fruit
1/2	cup low-sugar strawberry jam

In 1-cup glass measuring cup, sprinkle gelatin over 1/2 cup buttermilk. Let sit 1 minute to soften. Microwave on High for 2 minutes, stir to dissolve gelatin.

Use food processor or blender to process gelatin mixture, remaining buttermilk, sugar, peel, strawberry extract and lemon juice until blended. Add cottage cheese and process until smooth, scraping sides. With machine running, drop in 1 cup of strawberries and process just until small pieces of strawberries remain; scrape sides and pour into cooled crust. Cover with plastic wrap without wrap touching cake. Chill at least 3 hours or overnight until firm.

To serve, use a sharp knife to loosen sides of cake from pan. Remove sides and leaving cake on pan bottom, set on plate. Slice strawberries, peel and thinly slice kiwi. Arrange fruit on top of cake. Use blueberries to fill empty spots on top of cheesecake. Heat jam in microwave on High for 30 seconds; stir and spread over fruit arranged on top of cake. Serve or refrigerate until ready to serve.

KATHY'S CHEESECAKE

EVERY MOUTHFUL IS A CREAMY DELIGHT!
Prep time: 10 min   Bake time: 2 hrs   Chill time: Overnight
Serves: 8   Serving size: 1 Slice, 1/8 Portion
Exchanges: 1/2 Starch and 2 Skim milk (2 Carbohydrate Choices)
Analysis per serving: 213 Calories, 29 g Carbohydrate, 18 g Protein,
2 g Fat, 60 mg Cholesterol, 202 mg Sodium, 1 g Fiber

1/2	cup graham cracker crumbs
1	8-ounce package nonfat cream cheese, softened
2	cups nonfat ricotta cheese
1	tsp lemon juice
1	tsp vanilla extract
1	Tbs cornstarch
1/4	cup sugar
2	large eggs or 1/2 cup egg substitute
1	tsp dried lemon peel or grated fresh lemon peel
1 1/2	cups YOGURT CHEESE (page 83)
1/2	cup low-sugar jam of your choice
1	cup fresh fruit, washed & sliced

Preheat oven 350°F. Spray an 8-inch springform pan with cooking spray. Sprinkle bottom and sides of pan with graham cracker crumbs. Set aside. Have 13x9x2-inch pan ready.

Use food processor or blender to process cream cheese, ricotta, lemon juice, vanilla, cornstarch, sugar, eggs and peel; process until smooth, scraping sides. Add yogurt cheese and pulse and scrape sides 2 times until well combined; do not over process. Pour into prepared pan; place in oven. Put 13x9x2-inch pan on shelf below cake and fill with about 1-inch of boiling water. (This will prevent cheesecake from cracking.) Bake 55 to 60 minutes or until puffed and lightly browned. Leave cake in oven; turn off oven and leave door ajar about 1-inch for 1 hour. Remove from oven; cool.

Cover and refrigerate overnight. Before serving, run a sharp knife around sides of cake to loosen. Remove sides from pan and leaving cake on pan bottom, place on serving plate. If desired, arrange fruit decoratively on top. Microwave jam on High for 30 seconds; stir; spread over fruit to seal fruit or top with a fruit topping of your choice such as TEMPTING BLUEBERRY TOPPING (page 81).

MINI CHEESECAKES

A TERRIFIC WAY TO ENTERTAIN WITH CHEESECAKE
Prep time: 10 min   Bake time: 15 min   Chill time: 2 hrs
Makes: 4 dozen   Serving size: 3 Cakes, 1/16 Portion
Exchanges: 1 Skim milk (1 Carbohydrate Choice)
Analysis per serving: 106 Calories, 15 g Carbohydrate, 9 g Protein,
1 g Fat, 30 mg Cholesterol, 101 mg Sodium, 0 g Fiber

Prepare as directed in KATHY'S CHEESECAKE (page 92) but pour batter
in paper-lined mini muffin pans.

Bake at 350°F for 15 to 20 minutes or until puffed and lightly browned.
Remove from oven and cool on racks for at least 30 minutes.

Carefully remove from pans and cool completely on racks. Spoon fruit
topping of your choice, such as TEMPTING BLUEBERRY TOPPING
(page 81), on each mini cheesecake. Store covered in refrigerator.

❖ There is no need for water bath since they are so small.

PUMPKIN SWIRL CHEESECAKE

A NICE CHANGE FROM THE TRADITIONAL PUMPKIN PIE
Prep time: 10 min   Bake time 3 hrs   Chill time: 4 hrs
Serves: 10   Serving size: 1 Slice, 1/10 Portion
Exchanges: 1 Fruit, 1 Skim milk and 1 Fat (2 Carbohydrate Choices)
Analysis per serving: 200 Calories, 23 g Carbohydrate, 16 g Protein,
5 g Fat, 68 mg Cholesterol, 210 mg Sodium, 2 g Fiber

1	baked **OATMEAL CRUST** (page 181) in 9-inch springform pan
1	8-ounce package nonfat cream cheese, softened
2	cups nonfat ricotta cheese
1/4	cup sugar
3	large eggs or 3/4 cup egg substitute
1	tsp vanilla extract
1	Tbs cornstarch
1	cup **YOGURT CHEESE** (page 83)
1	cup canned or fresh pumpkin
3/4	tsp cinnamon
1/4	tsp nutmeg
1/2	tsp maple extract

Preheat oven 350°F. Prepare OATMEAL CRUST according to directions.

In food processor or blender or with mixer, combine cream cheese, ricotta cheese, sugar, eggs, vanilla, cornstarch and yogurt cheese until smooth, scraping sides occasionally. Remove 2 cups of mixture and set aside. Add pumpkin, spices and extract to mixture in food processor. Process until combined. Scrape sides and pour half of pumpkin mixture onto prepared crust. Pour half of plain mixture over pumpkin mixture. Repeat layers. Gently cut through batter with knife for a marbled effect. Be sure not to cut into crust.

Put filled pan in oven. Put 13x9x2-inch pan on shelf below and fill with boiling water to measure about 1-inch. (This helps to prevent cheesecake from cracking.) Bake 55 to 60 minutes. Shut off oven and leave cake in closed oven for 2 hours. Remove pans from oven and let pie cool before covering with plastic wrap. Refrigerate at least 4 hours or overnight.

To serve, use a sharp knife to loosen cake from pan. Remove sides and leaving cake on pan bottom, place on serving plate.

PINEAPPLE CHEESEPIE

SPLURGE! IT'S LOW-FAT!
Prep time: 10 min   Bake time: 30 min   Chill time: 4 hrs
Serves: 8   Serving size: 1 Slice, 1/8 Portion
Exchanges: 1 Skim milk (1 Carbohydrate Choice)
Analysis per serving: 88 Calories, 11 g Carbohydrate, 8 g Protein,
1 g Fat, 21 mg Cholesterol, 127 mg Sodium, 0 g Fiber

1	**20-ounce can juice-packed crushed pineapple**
1	**envelope unflavored gelatin**
2	**large egg whites, at room temperature**
1	**large egg yolk**
2	**cups nonfat ricotta cheese**
1	**tsp vanilla extract**
1	**tsp lemon juice**
1/2	**tsp dried lemon peel or grated fresh lemon peel**
1/4	**cup sugar**
1/4	**tsp salt**
Cinnamon	

Preheat oven 350°F. Have a 9-inch pie plate ready.

Drain pineapple over a 1-cup glass measuring cup to measure 1/2 cup juice. Set aside drained pineapple. Sprinkle gelatin over juice. Let sit 5 minutes to soften.

In medium bowl, use electric mixer at high speed to beat egg whites until stiff when lifted with a rubber spatula. In food processor or blender, combine egg yolk, reserved pineapple, ricotta and gelatin. Process until smooth; scrape sides and add vanilla, juice, peel, sugar and salt. Process until blended, scraping sides. Use a rubber spatula to gently fold cheese mixture into beaten whites until no white streaks remain. Pour into pie pan, sprinkle with cinnamon.

Bake 30 to 40 minutes or until firm and knife inserted in center comes out clean. Cool on rack. Refrigerate at least 4 hours or overnight before serving.

APPEALING
APPLE CHEESECAKE

IF YOU LOVE CHEESECAKE AND APPLES, YOU'LL LOVE THIS RECIPE
Prep time: 10 min   Bake time: 2 hrs   Chill time: 8 hrs
Serves: 8   Serving size: 1 Slice, 1/8 Portion
Exchanges: 2 Skim milk, 1/2 Fruit and 1 Fat (2 Carbohydrate Choices)
Analysis per serving: 242 Calories, 30 g Carbohydrate, 18 g Protein,
5 g Fat, 32 mg Cholesterol, 296 mg Sodium, 1 g Fiber

Crust

1/2	cup graham cracker crumbs
1/2	tsp cinnamon
1/4	tsp nutmeg
1	Tbs olive or canola oil

Filling

1/2	cup sugar
1/2	tsp cinnamon
2 1/2	cups nonfat ricotta cheese
1/2	cup buttermilk
1/4	cup all-purpose flour
1	8-ounce package nonfat cream cheese, softened
1/2	tsp dried lemon peel or grated fresh lemon peel
2	tsp vanilla extract
1/2	tsp almond extract
2	large egg whites
1	large egg
2	medium Rome apples, peeled, cored & cut into eighths
3	Tbs sliced almonds

Preheat oven 325°F. Spray an 8-inch springform pan with cooking spray.

In a small bowl, combine crust ingredients until well blended. Pat onto bottom and part-way up sides of prepared pan, set aside. Have a 13x9x2-inch pan ready.

Use food processor to process sugar, cinnamon, ricotta, buttermilk, flour, cream cheese, peel, extracts, whites and egg until smooth, about 1 minute; scrape sides and process 30 seconds or until well blended. With machine running, drop in apple pieces and process, scraping sides, just until small pieces of apple remain in batter. Pour cheese mixture into prepared pan and place in oven. On shelf below, place larger pan and carefully fill with hot water. (This will prevent the cheesecake from cracking.)

Bake for 1 hour. Carefully remove cheesecake from oven and sprinkle with sliced almonds. Return to oven and bake an additional 10 minutes. Shut off oven, keep door ajar 1-inch and leave in oven for 30 minutes. Remove cake and waterbath from oven and cool cheesecake on rack for 30 minutes. Cover and chill at least 8 hours before serving.

To serve, use a sharp knife to loosen cake from pan. Remove sides and leaving cake on pan bottom, place on serving plate.

SLIMMING CHEESECAKE

YOU WON'T FEEL GUILTY ENJOYING THIS CHEESECAKE
Prep time: 10 min   Bake time: 35 min   Chill time: 4 hrs
Makes: 16   Serving size: 1 Piece, 1/16 Portion
Exchanges: 1 Lean meat
Analysis per serving: .42 Calories, 4 g Carbohydrate, 6 g Protein,
0 g Fat, 0 mg Cholesterol, 60 mg Sodium, 0 mg Fiber

1	**cup nonfat cottage cheese**
1	**cup nonfat ricotta cheese**
2	**large eggs or 1/2 cup egg substitute**
4	**Tbs nonfat dry milk powder, divided**
2	**Tbs sugar**
1	**tsp vanilla extract**
1/2	**tsp dried lemon peel or grated fresh lemon peel**
2	**large egg whites, at room temperature**
1/4	**tsp cream of tartar**
1/2	**cup low-sugar jam of your choice (optional)**

Preheat oven 350°F. Spray an 8-inch square pan with cooking spray.

In food processor or blender, combine cottage cheese, ricotta cheese, eggs, 2 Tbs dry milk powder, sugar, vanilla and lemon peel. Process until smooth, scraping sides.   Set aside.

In medium bowl, beat egg whites and cream of tartar at high speed of electric mixer until foamy. Gradually beat in remaining 2 Tbs dry milk powder, scraping sides occasionally. Continue beating at high speed until soft peaks form when lifted with rubber spatula. Pour cheese mixture over beaten egg whites and use a rubber spatula to gently combine until no white streaks remain. Pour mixture into prepared pan.

Bake about 35 minutes or until top is browned and pick inserted in center comes out clean. Cool on rack about 1 hour. If desired, microwave jam on High for 30 seconds; stir, spread on top of cheesecake or serve plain with fruit on the side. Refrigerate, covered, at least 4 hours before cutting into 16 squares.

LAYERED
CHEESECAKE SQUARES

A DELICIOUS CHEESECAKE WITH A TASTY YOGURT TOPPING
Prep time: 5 min   Bake time: 30 min   Chill time: 4 hrs
Makes: 16 Squares   Serving size: 1 Square, 1/16 Portion
Exchanges: 1/2 Skim milk (1 Carbohydrate Choice)
Analysis per serving: 58 Calories, 7 g Carbohydrate, 5 g Protein,
1 g Fat, 18 mg Cholesterol, 45 mg Sodium, 0 g Fiber

2	cups nonfat cottage cheese
1/4	cup whole-wheat flour
2	large eggs or 1/2 cup egg substitute
1	Tbs lemon juice
1/4	cup sugar
1	tsp dried lemon peel or grated fresh lemon peel
1/2	cup plain nonfat yogurt
2	Tbs low-sugar jam of your choice

Preheat oven 325°F. Spray an 8-inch square pan with cooking spray.

In food processor or blender, combine cottage cheese, flour, eggs, juice, sugar and peel; process until smooth, scraping sides occasionally. Pour into prepared pan and bake about 25 minutes or until firm.

Meanwhile, in a small bowl, combine yogurt and jam until well blended.

Remove cheesecake from oven and immediately spread with yogurt mixture to cover completely. Return to oven; bake 5 minutes more. Remove from oven; cool on rack for 1 hour. Refrigerate, covered, at least 4 hours before cutting into squares.

CHEESY JAM SQUARES

Crust

2	**Tbs brown sugar**
3	**Tbs olive or canola oil**
1/2	**cup old-fashioned oats**
1/2	**cup whole-wheat flour**
1/4	**cup chopped nuts**

Preheat oven 350°F. Spray an 8-inch square pan with cooking spray.

In medium bowl, combine sugar and oil until well blended; stir in oatmeal, flour and nuts until crumbly. Reserve 1/2 cup. Press remaining mixture onto bottom of pan. Bake 8 to 10 minutes; set aside to cool.

Filling

1	**8-ounce package nonfat cream cheese**
2	**Tbs sugar**
1	**Tbs lemon juice**
2	**Tbs skim milk**
1/2	**tsp vanilla extract**
1	**large egg or 1/4 cup egg substitute**
3	**Tbs low-sugar raspberry jam**

In food processor, blender or with mixer, combine cream cheese and sugar until smooth. Add lemon juice, milk, vanilla and egg; process until smooth, scraping sides occasionally. Spread mixture over baked crust. Microwave jam on High for about 30 seconds; stir. Dribble melted jam over cheese mixture. Swirl with knife. Be sure not to cut into crust; sprinkle with reserved crumb mixture.

Bake 25 minutes or until firm and knife inserted in center comes out clean. Cool on rack. Refrigerate at least 2 hours before cutting into 16 squares.

PINEAPPLE CHEESECAKE SQUARES

A WONDERFUL AND PRETTY DESSERT FOR POTLUCKS AND REUNIONS
Prep time: 15 min   Bake time: 25 min   Chill time: 4 hrs
Makes: 24 Squares   Serving size: 1 Square, 1/24 Portion
Exchanges: 1 Starch (1 Carbohydrate Choice)
Analysis per serving: 93 Calories, 16 g Carbohydrate, 4 g Protein,
1 g Fat, 2 mg Cholesterol, 104 mg Sodium, 0 g Fiber

Crust

1 1/2	cups graham cracker crumbs
1/4	tsp nutmeg
1/2	tsp cinnamon
2	Tbs honey
1 1/2	Tbs olive or canola oil

Preheat oven 350°F. Spray a 13x9x2-inch pan with cooking spray. In medium bowl, use a fork to blend all ingredients. Press firmly onto bottom of prepared pan; set aside.

Filling

1	8-ounce package nonfat cream cheese, softened
1/4	cup sugar
5	large egg whites
1	6-ounce can (2/3 cup) unsweetened pineapple juice
1	cup nonfat ricotta cheese or cottage cheese
1	tsp vanilla extract

In food processor or blender or with electric mixer, combine all ingredients until smooth, scraping sides. Pour over crust; bake 25 to 30 minutes or until center is set. Cool on rack about 30 minutes.

Topping

1	20-ounce can juice-packed crushed pineapple
1-2	Tbs water
1/4	cup flour
1/4	cup sugar

Drain pineapple into a 4-cup glass measuring cup and add enough water to measure 1 cup; reserve crushed pineapple. Use a whisk or a fork to mix in flour and sugar until smooth. Microwave on High 2 minutes, stir, and microwave another 2 minutes, stirring every minute, or until thickened. Stir in reserved crushed pineapple, When cool, spread pineapple mixture over cooled cheesecake. Cover loosely and refrigerate about 4 hours or overnight. Cut into 2-inch squares to serve.

Coffee Cakes

Coffee cakes are wonderful with a cup of coffee or tea, delicious as an addition to breakfast, marvelous with brunch and great as a snack.

Most coffee cakes are easy and quick to prepare and many contain some sort of fruit or nuts. The coffee cakes in this book are so easy to prepare that preparing one for a gift is a snap and will be greatly appreciated by the recipient.

Coffee cakes can be baked and frozen for up to 3 months. Defrost at room temperature or unwrap and place on a paper plate to defrost in the microwave. These particular cakes are similar to muffins, scones and quick breads and should not be overmixed or the coffee cake will be tough. Mix ingredients just until blended. They can be prepared and baked in an 8- or 9-inch pan or an oblong or bundt or tube pan according to the recipe.

If baking coffee cake in a glass or Pyrex baking dish, lower oven temperature by 25°.

The coffee cakes in the DIABETIC GOODIE BOOK are reduced in fat, sugar and salt. A small amount of sugar is used in each recipe along with fruit or fruit juice for flavor, moisture and natural sweetness.

APPLE CRUMB COFFEE CAKE

A CHOPPED RIPE PEAR CAN BE SUBSTITUTED
Prep time: 10 min   Baking time: 30 min
Serves: 9   Serving size: 1 Piece, 1/9 Portion
Exchanges: 1 Starch, 1/2 Fruit and 1 1/2 Fat (2 Carbohydrate Choices)
Analysis per serving: 195 Calories, 26 g Carbohydrate, 4 g Protein,
9 g Fat, 24 mg Cholesterol, 190 mg Sodium, 2 g Fiber

3/4	cup whole-wheat flour
3/4	cup all-purpose flour
1	tsp baking powder
1/2	tsp baking soda
1/4	cup sugar
1/4	tsp salt
1	tsp dried lemon peel or grated fresh lemon peel
1	medium apple, peel, cored & chopped
1/4	cup olive or canola oil
3/4	cup skim milk
1	large egg or 1/4 cup egg substitute
1/2	tsp vanilla extract
1/4	cup chopped walnuts
1/2	tsp cinnamon
1/4	tsp nutmeg
1	Tbs brown sugar

Preheat oven 350°F. Spray an 9-inch round or square baking pan with cooking spray. In medium bowl, combine flours, baking powder, baking soda, salt, sugar and peel until blended. Stir in chopped apple until apple is coated with flour mixture.

In small bowl, use a whisk or fork to blend oil, milk, egg and vanilla. Stir wet ingredients into apple mixture just until moistened; do not over mix. Spread batter into prepared pan. In same small bowl, combine walnuts, cinnamon, nutmeg and brown sugar; sprinkle over batter. Bake 30 minutes or until cake is browned and pick inserted in center comes out clean. Cool about 10 minutes on rack before serving. May be served warm or at room temperature. Refrigerate after 2 days or freeze up to 3 months.

If desired, spoon batter into an 9-inch round pan which has been sprayed with cooking spray and arrange another apple, peeled, cored and thinly sliced in a circular pattern on top of batter. Sprinkle with walnut mixture. Bake as directed.

BANANA DATE CRUMB COFFEE CAKE

SO MOIST & TASTY — GREAT FOR A CROWD
Prep time: 10 min   Bake time: 20 min
Serves: 24   Serving size:1 Piece, 1/24 Portion
Exchanges: 1 Starch, 1/2 Fruit and 1 Fat (1 Carbohydrate Choice)
Analysis per serving: 147 Calories, 21 g Carbohydrate, 3 g Protein,
6 g Fat, 0 mg Cholesterol, 80 mg Sodium, 2 g Fiber

1 1/2	cups all-purpose flour
1 1/2	cups whole-wheat flour
1	tsp baking soda
2	tsp baking powder
2	Tbs sugar
1	cup chopped dates
1/2	cup olive or canola oil
1/2	cup mashed ripe banana (1 medium)
3/4	cup egg substitute
1	tsp vanilla extract
1	cup orange juice
1	tsp dried orange peel or grated fresh orange peel

Preheat oven 350°F. Spray 13x9x2-inch baking pan with cooking spray.
In large bowl, combine flours, baking soda, baking powder and sugar until
blended. Stir in dates until coated with flour mixture.   In small bowl, use a
whisk or a fork to combine oil, mashed banana, egg substitute, vanilla,
juice and peel until well mixed. Stir wet ingredients into flour mixture and
mix with wooden spoon or rubber spatula until well blended.   Spoon batter
into prepared pan and sprinkle with topping.

Topping

1/4	cup chopped walnuts
1/4	cup flaked coconut
1	Tbs brown sugar
1/2	tsp cinnamon
1/4	tsp nutmeg

In a small bowl, combine all topping ingredients and sprinkle evenly over
batter. Bake 25 to 30 minutes or until browned and pick inserted in center
comes out clean. Cool on rack at least 10 minutes before serving. May
be served warm or at room temperature. Refrigerate after 2 days or
freeze up to 3 months.

BERRY COFFEE CAKE

USE FRESH OR FROZEN RASPBERRIES, BLACKBERRIES OR BLUEBERRIES
Prep time: 10 min   Baking time: 30 min
Serves: 9   Serving size: 1 Piece, 1/9 Portion
Exchanges: 1 Starch, 1/2 Fruit and 1 Fat (2 Carbohydrate Choices)
Analysis per serving: 162 Calories, 24 g Carbohydrate, 4 g Protein,
5 g Fat, 24 mg Cholesterol, 156 mg Sodium, 3 g Fiber

3/4	cup whole-wheat flour
3/4	cup all-purpose flour
3	Tbs nonfat dry milk powder or buttermilk powder
3	Tbs brown sugar
1 1/2	tsp baking powder
1/4	tsp salt
3	Tbs olive or canola oil
3/4	cup orange juice
1	large egg or 1/4 cup egg substitute
2	tsp dried orange peel or grated fresh orange peel
1/2	tsp vanilla extract
1	cup fresh or frozen raspberries, blueberries or blackberries
1	Tbs sugar

Preheat oven 350°F. Spray a 9-inch round or square baking pan with cooking spray.

In large bowl, sift flours, dry milk or buttermilk, brown sugar, baking powder and salt. If whole-wheat particles remain in sifter, just add grains to flour mixture. Use a pastry blender, fork or two knives scissor-fashion to cut in oil until mixture is crumbly; set aside.

 In small bowl, use a whisk or fork to combine juice, egg, peel and vanilla until blended. Stir wet ingredients into dry ingredients and mix just until blended; do not overmix. Spoon batter into prepared pan.

In same small bowl, combine berries and sugar until berries are coated. Sprinkle berries over batter. Bake 30 to 35 minutes or until cake is browned and pick inserted in center comes out clean. Cool on rack about 10 minutes before serving.

May be served warm or at room temperature. Refrigerate after 2 days or freeze up to 3 months.

BUTTERMILK
SPICE COFFEE CAKE

AN EGGLESS CAKE USING COCOA POWDER AS A SEASONING
Prep time: 10 min   Baking time: 30 min
Serves: 9   Serving size: 1 Piece, 1/9 Portion
Exchanges: 1 Starch and 2 Fat (2 Carbohydrate Choices)
Analysis per serving: 190 Calories, 26 g Carbohydrate, 4 g Protein,
9 g Fat, 1 mg Cholesterol, 102 mg Sodium, 2 g Fiber

3/4	cup whole-wheat flour
3/4	cup all-purpose flour
1/4	cup sugar
1/4	cup olive or canola oil
1/2	tsp baking soda
1/4	tsp baking powder
2	tsp cinnamon
1 1/2	tsp cocoa
1/2	tsp nutmeg
1/8	tsp cloves
1/4	cup raisins
1	cup buttermilk
1/4	cup chopped nuts

Preheat oven 350°F. Spray 9-inch square baking pan with cooking spray.

In large bowl, combine flours, and sugar. With pastry blender, fork or two knives scissor-fashion, cut in oil until mixture is crumbly. Measure out 1/2 cup of crumb mixture and set aside.

To remaining crumb mixture, add baking soda, baking powder, cinnamon, cocoa, nutmeg, cloves and raisins; mix well. Make a well in dry ingredients and add buttermilk. Use a wooden spoon or rubber spatula to combine just until moistened; do not overmix. Spoon batter into prepared pan.

Stir nuts into reserved crumb mixture and sprinkle over batter. Bake 30 to 35 minutes or until browned and pick inserted in center comes out clean. Cool on rack 10 minutes before serving. Serve warm or at room temperature. Can be frozen up to 3 months.

NUTTY RASPBERRY COFFEE CAKE

THE RASPBERRIES ADD SUCH PRETTY COLOR AND FLAVOR
Prep time: 10 min   Baking time: 40 min
Serves: 9   Serving size: 1 Piece, 1/9 Portion
Exchanges: 1 Starch and 1 Fat (1 Carbohydrate Choice)
Analysis per serving: 126 Calories, 19 g Carbohydrate, 3 g Protein,
4 g Fat, 24 mg Cholesterol, 67 mg Sodium, 2 g Fiber

1	cup fresh raspberries
1	Tbs brown sugar
1/2	cup whole-wheat flour
1/2	cup all-purpose flour
1/4	cup sugar
1/2	tsp baking powder
1/4	tsp baking soda
1/2	cup plain nonfat yogurt
2	Tbs olive or canola oil
1	tsp vanilla extract
1	large egg or 1/4 cup egg substitute
1	Tbs sliced almonds
	Confectioners' sugar (optional)

Preheat oven 350°F. Spray 9-inch round or square baking pan with cooking spray.

In a small bowl, combine raspberries and brown sugar; set aside.

In a large bowl, combine flours, sugar, baking powder and baking soda until blended.

In another small bowl, combine yogurt, oil, vanilla and egg until well blended. Stir wet ingredients into dry ingredients just until moistened; do not overmix. Set aside about 1/2 cup of batter. Spoon remaining batter into prepared pan; spread evenly. Sprinkle reserved raspberries evenly over batter. Spoon remaining batter over raspberries spreading to cover top of raspberries; sprinkle with almonds.

Bake for 40 minutes or until browned and pick inserted in center comes out clean. Cool on rack. If desired, sprinkle with confectioners' sugar before serving. Serve warm or at room temperature. Store, covered, at room temperature up to 2 days. Can be frozen up to 3 months.

PINEAPPLE COFFEE CAKE

A COFFEE CAKE WITH A TROPICAL FLAVOR
Prep time: 10 min   Baking time: 25 min
Serves: 21   Serving size: 1 Piece, 1/21 Portion
Exchanges: 1 Starch and 1 Fat (1 Carbohydrate Choice)
Analysis per serving: 110 Calories, 17 g Carboyhdrate, 2 g Protein,
4 g Fat, 0 mg Cholesterol, 54 mg Sodium, 1 g Fiber

1	20-ounce can juice-packed crushed pineapple
1	cup whole-wheat flour
1	cup all-purpose flour
2	Tbs sugar
1/4	tsp salt
2	tsp baking powder
6	Tbs olive or canola oil, divided
1	large egg or 1/4 cup egg substitute
1/4	cup brown sugar
1/4	cup sifted all-purpose flour

Preheat oven 400°F. Spray 11x7-inch baking pan with cooking spray.
Drain pineapple; reserve juice.

In a large bowl, combine flours, sugar, salt and baking powder.

In small bowl, combine 4 Tbs oil, egg and 1/3 cup reserved pineapple
juice until well blended. Stir wet ingredients into dry ingredients until well
mixed. Batter will be very thick. Press into prepared pan .

In small bowl, use a fork to combine 2 Tbs oil, brown sugar and 1/4 cup
flour until crumbly. Stir in reserved crushed, drained pineapple and mix
well. Spoon over batter.

Bake 25 to 30 minutes or until browned and pick inserted in center comes
out clean. Cool on rack 10 minutes before serving. Serve warm or at
room temperature. Refrigerate after 2 days. Can be frozen up to 3
months.

❖ If using a glass baking pan, reduce oven temperature to 375°F. Bake
30 minutes or until browned and pick inserted in center comes out clean.

SPEEDY CHOCOLATE COFFEE CAKE

ALMOST LIKE EATING A BROWNIE
Prep time: 10 min   Bake time: 35 min
Serves: 9   Serving size: 1 Piece, 1/9 Portion
Exchanges: 1 Starch, 1/2 Fruit and 2 Fat (2 Carbohydrate Choices)
Analysis per serving: 206 Calories, 27 g Carbohydrate, 6 g Protein,
9 g Fat, 1 mg Cholesterol, 195 mg Sodium, 3 g Fiber

3/4	cup whole-wheat flour
3/4	cup all-purpose flour
2	tsp baking powder
1/4	tsp salt
1/4	cup sugar
2	Tbs brown sugar
1/4	cup cocoa
1	cup plain nonfat yogurt
1/4	cup olive or canola oil
1/2	cup egg substitute
1	tsp vanilla
1/4	cup chopped nuts

Preheat oven 350°F. Spray 9-inch square baking pan with cooking spray.

In large bowl, combine flours, baking powder, salt, sugar, brown sugar, cocoa, yogurt, oil, egg substitute and vanilla. Stir with wooden spoon or rubber spatula, about 1 minute, until well blended. Spoon into prepared pan and sprinkle with nuts.

Bake 35 to 40 minutes or until browned and pick inserted in center comes out clean. Cool about 10 minutes before serving. Serve warm or at room temperature. Can be frozen up to 3 months.

STREUSEL COFFEE CAKE

AN ELEGANT COFFEE CAKE WITH A SURPRISE IN THE MIDDLE
Prep time: 10 min   Baking time: 55 min
Serves: 20   Serving size: 1 Piece, 1/20 Portion
Exchanges: 1 Starch, 1 Fruit and 1/2 Fat (2 Carbohydrate Choices)
Analysis per serving: 147 Calories, 25 g Carbohydrate, 4 g Protein,
4 g Fat, 0 mg Cholesterol, 108 mg Sodium, 2 g Fiber

Streusel

1	**Tbs olive or canola oil**
1/4	**cup brown sugar**
1/2	**tsp cinnamon**
1/2	**cup raisins**

In small bowl, combine all ingredients; set aside.

1 1/2	**cups whole-wheat flour**
1 1/2	**cups all-purpose flour**
1/3	**cup sugar**
2	**tsp baking powder**
3/4	**tsp baking soda**
1/4	**cup chopped dried apricots**
1 1/2	**cups plain nonfat yogurt**
1/4	**cup olive or canola oil**
3/4	**cup egg substitute**
2	**tsp dried lemon peel or grated fresh lemon peel**
1	**tsp vanilla extract**
	Confectioners' sugar

Preheat oven 350°F. Spray a 12-cup bundt cake pan with cooking spray.
In large bowl, combine flours, sugar, baking powder, baking soda and
chopped apricots.

In small bowl, combine yogurt, oil, egg substitute, lemon peel and extract
until blended. Using a rubber spatula or wooden spoon, gently add wet
ingredients to dry ingredients until thoroughly blended; do not over mix.
Spoon half of batter into prepared pan. Sprinkle with reserved Streusel
mixture. Spoon remaining batter over Streusel.

Bake 55 to 60 minutes or until browned and pick inserted in center comes
out clean. Cool on wire rack for 10 minutes. Invert onto serving plate;
cool completely on rack. Sprinkle with confectioners' sugar before serving.

MIXED BERRY COFFEE CAKE

SIMPLE TO PREPARE AND SCRUMPTIOUS
Prep Time: 10 min   Bake Time: 50 min
Serves: 12   Serving size: 1 Wedge, 1/12 Serving
Exchanges: 1 Starch, 1/2 Fruit, 1/2 Fat (1 Carbohydrate Choice)
Analysis per serving: 124 Calories, 22 g Carbohydrate, 4 g Protein,
3 g Fat, 0 mg Cholesterol, 135 mg Sodium, 3 g Fiber

3/4	cup whole-wheat flour
3/4	cup all-purpose flour
2	tsp baking powder
1/2	tsp baking soda
4	large egg whites or 1/2 cup egg substitute
2	Tbs sugar
2/3	cup unsweetened applesauce
1/4	cup nonfat plain yogurt
1	tsp dried or freshly grated lemon peel
2	cups assorted fresh or frozen berries (blueberries, blackberries, raspberries)
1/4	cup all-purpose flour
3	Tbs brown sugar
2	Tbs olive or canola oil

Preheat oven 350°F. Spray a 10-inch springform pan with cooking spray.

In a small bowl, combine flours, baking powder and baking soda. In a medium bowl, use a whisk to blend egg whites, sugar, applesauce, yogurt and lemon peel until well mixed. Add flour mixture to wet ingredients just until blended. Spread into prepared pan. Sprinkle mixed berries on top of batter.

In same small bowl, combine 1/4 cup flour and brown sugar. Stir in oil until blended. Sprinkle mixture evenly over berries. Bake 50 to 55 minutes until pick inserted in center comes out clean. Cool 20 minutes before serving.

To serve, loosen sides of cake with a knife and removes sides of pan; place on serving plate. The cooled coffee cake can be frozen, well wrapped, up to 3 months.

Fruit Desserts

There are a variety of fruit-based desserts in this section. Some are quick, less than 5 minutes to fix, while others require more lengthy preparation and cooking time.

The recipes range from easy and basic to elegant. SPEEDY FRUIT CRISP will please kids, and you can choose almost any fruit you want for it. APPLE NUT TORTE or BAKED MERINGUE PEARS are lovely ways to end a dinner party with friends. Look for frozen desserts as well as baked crisps.

Made ahead, many of these recipes are also perfect lunch-packers and snacks. The LIGHT & FRUITY SHAKE is great for breakfast!

For your convenience, a fruit chart is included in this book on pages 239-241. Items listed by fruit include availability, peak season, description, buying and storing hints and specifics about each fruit.

MICROWAVE APPLESAUCE

WELL WORTH THE EFFORT
Prep time: 10 min   Cook time: 20 min
Serves: 6   Serving size: 1/2 Cup
Exchanges: 1 1/3 Fruit (1 Carbohydrate Choice)
Analysis per serving: 80 Calories, 20 g Carbohydrate, 0 g Protein,
0 g Fat, 0 mg Cholesterol, 0 mg Sodium, 2 g Fiber

6	**Golden Delicious apples (about 8 cups), peeled, cored & sliced**
1/4	**cup water**
1	**Tbs sugar**
2	**tsp lemon juice**
3/4	**tsp cinnamon**
1/2	**tsp dried lemon peel or grated fresh lemon peel**

In a 3-quart microwavable bowl, combine apple slices and water. Cover and microwave on High for 15 minutes, stirring and rotating every 5 minutes or until apples are tender.

Stir in remaining ingredients. Let stand covered for 5 minutes, then mash or puree in food processor. Serve warm or chilled.

CHUNKY APPLESAUCE: Chop 1 peeled apple and mix with 1 Tbs of water in a small microwavable bowl. Cover and microwave for 3 minutes, stirring after 1 1/2 minutes or until apple chunks are tender. Add to mashed or pureed applesauce.

RASPBERRY APPLESAUCE

JUST SCRUMPTIOUS
Prep time: 10 min   Cook time: 20 min
Serves: 8   Serving size: 1/2 Cup
Exchanges: 1 Fruit (1 Carbohydrate Choice)
Analysis per serving: 68 Calories, 18 g Carbohydrate, 0 g Protein,
0 g Fat, 0 mg Cholesterol, 0 mg Sodium, 3 g Fiber

1   recipe MICROWAVE APPLESAUCE (page 114)
1   cup fresh or frozen unsweetened raspberries

Add 1 cup of fresh or natural frozen raspberries to MICROWAVE
APPLESAUCE immediately after removing applesauce from microwave.

Cover, let stand 5 minutes. Serve warm or chilled.

APPLE-BERRY-GURT DESSERT

A FAST-FIXING DESSERT THAT IS SO GOOD
Prep time: 5 min   Cook time: 30 min
Serves: 8   Serving size:1/2 Cup
Exchanges: 1 Fruit (1 Carbohydrate Choice)
Analysis per serving: 64 Calories, 15 g Carbohydrate, 2 g Protein,
0 g Fat, 1 mg Cholesterol, 16 mg Sodium, 2 g Fiber

2   cups unsweetened applesauce
1   cup plain nonfat yogurt
2   Tbs honey
1   cup fresh or frozen unsweetened raspberries

In a 4-cup measuring cup, combine applesauce, yogurt and honey until
blended. Gently stir in raspberries. Spoon into dessert dishes and
refrigerate about 30 minutes or until ready to serve. Refrigerate leftovers
covered.

APPLE NUT TORTE

SO SIMPLE AND SO SCRUMPTIOUS!
Prep time: 5 min   Bake time: 30 min
Serves: 8   Serving size: 1 Wedge, 1/8 Portion
Exchanges: 1 Fruit and 1/2 Fat (1 Carbohydrate Choice)
Analysis per serving: 83 Calories, 13 g Carbohydrate, 2 g Protein,
3 g Fat, 27 mg Cholesterol, 72 mg Sodium, 1 g Fiber

1/4	**cup chopped nuts**
1	**large egg**
1/4	**cup sugar**
1/4	**cup whole-wheat flour**
1 1/4	**tsp baking powder**
1 1/2	**cups apple, peeled, cored & chopped (1 large)**
1/2	**tsp vanilla extract**

Heat oven to 375°F. Spray an 8 or 9-inch pie pan with cooking spray.
Place nuts in prepared pan and toast nuts 3 to 5 minutes; cool.

In a small bowl, use electric mixer at medium speed to beat egg until
light and frothy. Gradually beat in sugar until thick, about 2 minutes;
scrape sides of bowl. Use a rubber spatula to stir flour, baking powder,
chopped apple, vanilla extract and toasted nuts into egg mixture; mix until
well blended.

Spoon into prepared pan and bake for 30 minutes or until browned. Cut in
wedges and serve warm with WHIPPED TOPPING (page 79) or lightly
sprinkled with confectioners' sugar.

SIMPLE BAKED APPLES

BAKE IN THE OVEN OR MICROWAVE IN HALF THE TIME
Prep time: 10 min   Bake time: 10 or 25 min
Serves: 4   Serving size: 1 Baked Apple
Exchanges: 1 1/2 Fruit (2 Carbohydrate Choices)
Analysis per serving: 95 Calories, 25 g Carbohydrate, 0 g Protein,
0 g Fat, 0 mg Cholesterol, 1 mg Sodium, 3 g Fiber

4	**medium Rome apples, washed**
2	**tsp lemon juice**
2	**tsp dried or freshly grated lemon peel**
2	**tsp cinnamon**
1	**tsp nutmeg**
2	**Tbs raisins (optional)**
1/2	**cup apple or appleblend juice**

Spray cooking spray in a casserole large enough to hold apples.

Using a vegetable peeler, peel about 1 inch of apple peel from top of each apple. Using end of peeler or a knife, cut around stem and remove stem and core with seeds.

Sprinkle the inside and peeled section of each apple with about 1/2 teaspoon lemon juice, 1/2 teaspoon lemon peel, 1/2 teaspoon cinnamon and 1/4 teaspoon nutmeg. If desired, stuff each apple with 1/2 tablespoon of raisins. Place seasoned apples in prepared casserole; pour juice over each apple, being sure that some juice goes into cavity of each apple. Cover.

To microwave: Cook on High 8 to 12 minutes, turning apples every 3 minutes and basting with juices in casserole until apples are tender. Let rest 10 minutes before serving.

To bake: Place covered casserole in preheated 400°F oven for 25 minutes, basting apples with cooking juices 2 or 3 times. Let rest 10 minutes before serving.

These apples are fantastic served cold or at room temperature. To serve, place in dessert bowl and spoon cooking juice over each apple.

FRUIT WITH YOGURT CREAM

WHEN YOU WANT A GREAT DESSERT REAL QUICK, THIS IS IT
Prep Time: 5 min   Cook Time: 0 min
Serves: 4   Serving size: 1/2 Cup
Exchanges: 1 Fruit (1 Carbohydrate Choice)
Analysis per serving: 46 Calories, 10 g Carbohydrate, 2 g Protein,
0 g Fat, 1 mg Cholesterol, 17 mg Sodium, 2 g Fiber

1/2	cup yogurt or YOGURT CHEESE (page 83)
1	tsp brown sugar
1	Tbs orange juice
1/8	tsp almond extract
1/2	tsp dried or freshly grated orange peel
1/4	tsp cinnamon
1/8	tsp nutmeg
2	cups washed and sliced fruit of your choice
1/4	cup sliced toasted almonds (optional)

In medium bowl, combine yogurt, brown sugar, orange juice, almond extract, orange peel, cinnamon and nutmeg until smooth and creamy. Stir in fruit until well coated with mixture. If desired, sprinkle with toasted almonds. Can be prepared, covered and refrigerated until ready to serve.

Suggested fruits: bananas, strawberries, fresh or canned peach slices or a mixture of fruits of your choice.

SPEEDY FRUIT CRISP

SO SIMPLE TO MAKE WITH YOUR FAVORITE FRUIT
Prep time: 10 min   Cook time: 30 min
Serves: 8   Serving size: 1/2 Cup
Exchanges: 1 Starch and 1 Fat (1 Carbohydrate Choice)
Analysis per serving: 128 Calories, 15 g Carbohydrate, 2 g Protein,
8 g Fat, 0 mg Cholesterol, 1 mg Sodium, 2 g Fiber

Filling

4	cups fruit of your choice (see below)
1	Tbs lemon juice
1	tsp dried lemon peel or grated fresh lemon peel
1	tsp sugar

Topping

1/4	cup whole-wheat flour
1/4	cup old-fashioned oats
1/4	cup chopped nuts
1/2	tsp cinnamon
1/2	tsp nutmeg
1	Tbs brown sugar
3	Tbs olive or canola oil

Spray an 8- or 9-inch glass pie plate or shallow casserole dish with cooking spray. In a large bowl, mix all filling ingredients and spoon into prepared pie plate or casserole. In same bowl, mix all topping ingredients and sprinkle over fruit filling.

To microwave: Microwave on High for 12 to 15 minutes, rotating every 4 minutes. Let stand for 15 minutes before serving.

To bake: Preheat oven 400°F. A metal pie plate can be used. Prepare as directed and bake for 30 to 40 minutes or until top is browned and fruit is tender. If desired, serve with WHIPPED TOPPING (page 79)or EASY FAT-FREE TOPPING (page 80).

❖ Suggested Fruits: 3-4 apples, peeled, cored and thinly sliced. 3-4 ripe pears, peeled, cored and thinly sliced. 6-8 medium ripe peaches, peeled, cored and thinly sliced. 2 cups strawberries hulled and sliced mixed with 2 cups rhubarb which has been washed and cut into 1-inch cubes. 4 medium bananas, peeled and thinly sliced. 6-8 medium ripe plums, cored and thinly sliced. 6-8 medium ripe nectarines, cored and thinly sliced. OR, use 2 16-ounce cans each of juice-packed fruit of your choice, and drain fruit before preparing filling.

BLUEBERRY NECTARINE CRISP

USE WHIPPED TOPPING (page79) or FAT-FREE WHIPPED TOPPING (page 80)
Prep time: 5 min   Cook time: 30 min or 12 min
Serves: 8   Serving size: 1/2 Cup
Exchanges: 1 Starch and 1 Fat (1 Carbohydrate Choice)
Analysis per serving: 130 Calories, 19 g Carbohydrate, 2 g Protein,
6 g Fat, 0 mg Cholesterol, 3 mg Sodium, 2 g Fiber

Filling

2	cups (1 pint) blueberries, washed & drained
2	medium ripe nectarines, washed, cored & sliced

Topping

1/4	cup all-purpose flour
1/4	cup whole-wheat flour
1/4	cup old-fashioned oats
2	Tbs brown sugar
1/2	tsp cinnamon
1/4	tsp nutmeg
3	Tbs olive or canola oil

Preheat oven to 400°F. Spray a quiche pan or shallow 2-quart casserole dish with cooking spray.

Place nectarine slices on bottom of prepared baking pan. Cover slices with blueberries.

In a small bowl, mix topping ingredients and sprinkle over fruits.

To Microwave: Microwave on High for 12 minutes, rotating every 4 minutes. Let stand for 15 minutes before serving.

To Bake: Bake for 20 to 25 minutes or until browned. Cool 15 minutes before serving.

PEACH MELBA PARFAIT

A COLORFUL FINISH TO A SIMPLE OR SPECIAL MEAL
Prep time: 10 min   Cook time: 30 min
Serves: 6   Serving size: 3/4 Cup
Exchanges: 1 Skim milk and 1 Fruit (1 Carbohydrate Choice)
Analysis per serving: 95 Calories, 21 g Carbohydrate, 4 g Protein,
0 g Fat, 0 mg Cholesterol, 45 mg Sodium, 1 g Fiber

3	**peaches, washed & thinly sliced**
2	**tsp lemon juice**
2	**cups plain nonfat yogurt**
1	**Tbs sugar**
1/2	**tsp vanilla extract**
1/4	**cup low-sugar raspberry jam**

In medium bowl, gently mix sliced peaches and lemon juice.

In another bowl, mix together yogurt, sugar and vanilla extract. Cover both dishes and refrigerate at least 30 minutes for flavors to blend.

To serve, use parfait dishes to layer peaches, yogurt mixture and raspberry jam; repeat, ending with jam.

❖ One 16-ounce can juice-packed sliced peaches, drained, can be substituted for fresh peaches. There is no need to mix canned sliced peaches with lemon juice. Proceed as directed.

PEACH SNOWCAPS

THEY RESEMBLE PORCUPINES
Prep time: 10 min   Bake time: 15 min
Serves: 4   Serving size: 1 Peach Half
Exchanges: 1 Starch (1 Carbohydrate Choice)
Analysis per serving: 92 Calories, 16 g Carbohydrate, 3 g Protein,
2 g Fat, 0 mg Cholesterol, 31 mg Sodium, 1 g Fiber

4	canned juice-packed peach halves
2	large egg whites, at room temperature
1/4	tsp almond extract
1/8	tsp cream of tartar
2	Tbs sugar
2	Tbs slivered almonds

Preheat oven to 325°F. Spray baking sheet with cooking spray. Dry peach halves with paper towels to assure that meringue will adhere. Place cut side down on prepared baking sheet.

In small bowl, beat egg whites, almond extract and cream of tartar with electric mixer at medium speed until foamy. Increase speed to high and gradually beat in sugar until stiff peaks form, scraping bowl occasionally. Spoon meringue over each peach half, covering completely. Stud each peach half with slivered almonds. Bake 15 to 20 minutes or until meringue is browned. Let stand 5 minutes before serving.

BAKED MERINGUE PEARS

A DIFFERENT WAY TO SERVE PEARS
Prep time: 15 min   Bake time: 25 min
Serves: 4   Serving size: 1/2 Pear
Exchanges: 1 Starch (1 Carbohydrate Choice)
Analysis per serving: 113 Calories, 19 g Carbohydrate, 1 g Protein,
0 g Fat, 0 mg Cholesterol, 14 mg Sodium, 2 g Fiber

2	large Anjou pears, peeled, halved lengthwise & cored
2	tsp sugar
2	tsp dried lemon peel or grated fresh lemon peel
1/4	cup dry vermouth
1	large egg white, at room temperature
1/8	tsp cream of tartar
2	Tbs confectioners' sugar
1/4	tsp almond extract

Arrange pears cut side up in baking dish sprayed with cooking spray. Sprinkle each half with 1/2 tsp sugar and 1/2 tsp lemon peel. Pour vermouth over pears and microwave on High for 15 minutes, rotating and basting every 5 minutes.

Preheat oven to 350°F. Spray baking sheet with cooking spray. With slotted spoon, transfer pear halves, cut side up to baking sheet. Reserve cooking liquid; set aside.

In a small bowl, beat egg white with electric mixer at medium speed until foamy, add cream of tartar and beat at high speed until soft peaks form. Gradually beat in confectioners' sugar and almond extract until whites are stiff, scraping bowl occasionally. Cover each pear completely with meringue. Bake 10 to 15 minutes or until meringue is brown.

While pears are baking, place reserved liquid in glass measuring cup and microwave on High for 2 minutes, stir cook on Medium/High until syrupy, about 2 minutes. Place pear halves on plates and spoon warm syrup over each pear half; serve warm or at room temperature.

BERRY BAKED PEARS

TOASTED NUTS AND BERRY TASTY PEARS — DELISH
Prep time: 5 min   Bake time: 35 min
Serves: 8   Serving size: 1 Pear Half
Exchanges: 1 Fruit and 1 Fat (1 Carbohydrate Choice)
Analysis per serving: 110 Calories, 18 g Carbohydrate, 2 g Protein,
4 g Fat, 2 mg Cholesterol, 9 mg Sodium, 3 g Fiber

4	pears, peeled, halved & cored
1/4	cup low-sugar raspberry jam
2	tsp lemon juice
1	tsp vanilla extract
1/3	cup sliced almonds
1	Tbs light margarine or light butter, cut into tiny pieces
1	cup plain nonfat yogurt (optional)

Preheat oven to 350°F. Spray a 9-inch pan or pie pan with cooking spray. Arrange pear halves, cut side down in pan.

In small bowl, mix together jam, lemon juice and vanilla and drizzle over pears. Sprinkle with almonds and dot with light margarine. Bake 35 to 40 minutes, basting 3 times, until pears are tender.

Let rest 15 minutes before serving. Serve warm or if desired, cold with yogurt. Store leftovers, covered, in refrigerator.

STRAWBERRY RHUBARB DESSERT

STRAWBERRIES ADD SWEETNESS AND COLOR TO TANGY RHUBARB
Prep time: 10 min   Cook time: 30 min
Serves: 8   Serving size: 1/2 Cup
Exchanges: 1 Fruit (1 Carbohydrate Choice)
Analysis per serving: 51 Calories, 12 g Carbohydrate, 1 g Protein,
0 g Fat, 0 mg Cholesterol, 4 mg Sodium, 2 g Fiber

1	pound fresh rhubarb stalks, washed & trimmed
3	Tbs sugar
1/2	tsp dried lemon peel or grated fresh lemon peel
1/2	tsp cinnamon
1/4	cup water
2	cups (1 pint) fresh strawberries, washed, hulled & halved
2	Tbs low-sugar strawberry jam

Cut rhubarb into 1-inch pieces; set aside. In a 4-cup glass measuring cup, mix together sugar, lemon peel, cinnamon and water. Microwave on High for 1 minute, stir and microwave for another minute until the sugar dissolves.

Add rhubarb, cover and microwave on Medium/High for 4 to 6 minutes, stirring every 2 minutes, until rhubarb is soft and tender.

Carefully stir strawberries and jam into rhubarb mixture until well mixed. Spoon into dessert dishes and refrigerate about 30 minutes before serving. If desired, serve with WHIPPED TOPPING (page 79) or EASY FAT-FREE TOPPING (page 80).

PINEAPPLE SHERBET

FAT-FREE AND SO GOOD
Prep time: 10 min   Freeze time: 90 min
Serves: 8   Serving size: 1/2 Cup
Exchanges: 1 Fruit (1 Carbohydrate Choice)
Analysis per serving: 45 Calories, 12 g Carbohydrate, 1 g Protein,
0 g Fat, 0 mg Cholesterol, 5 mg Sodium, 1 g Fiber

1	**20-ounce can juice-packed pineapple chunks**
1/4	**cup skim milk**

Drain pineapple, reserving juice. Place drained pineapple chunks on baking sheet with sides not touching. Put tray in freezer until chunks are hard, about 1 hour.

With machine running, gradually drop frozen chunks into food processor and process 1 minute; scrape sides. With machine running add reserved pineapple juice and milk. Process about 30 seconds, scraping sides, until mixture is smooth.

Pour into a 9-inch square pan and freeze about 1 hour until very firm. Remove from freezer and let stand about 10 minutes. Cut into squares and process in food processor until smooth, scraping sides occasionally. Serve immediately or spoon into a covered container and freeze up to 2 weeks. Remove from freezer about 15 minutes before serving to soften sherbet.

❖ One 16-ounce can of juice-packed peaches, apricots or pears, drained, (reserve juice) and cut into 1-inch chunks may be substituted. Add 1/2 of reserved juice along with the milk when processing.

If desired, 2 cups of any fresh washed fruit (peel, if necessary) may be used. Cut into chunks before freezing on baking sheet. Add 1/2 cup of fruit juice along with the milk when processing.

STRAWBERRY SORBET

FROZEN NATURAL STRAWBERRIES WILL REDUCE FREEZER TIME
Prep time: 10 min   Freeze time: 3 1/2 hrs
Serves: 8   Serving size: 1/2 Cup
Exchanges: 1 Fruit (1 Carbohydrate Choice)
Analysis per serving: 48 Calories, 12 g Carbohydrate, 0 g Protein,
0 g Fat, 0 mg Cholesterol, 1 mg Sodium, 1 g Fiber

2	cups (1 pint) strawberries, washed, drained & hulled
1	cup orange juice
1/4	cup sugar
1	cup water
2	Tbs lemon juice
1 1/2	tsp dried orange peel or grated fresh orange peel

In a food processor, combine strawberries, orange juice and sugar. Process until smooth, scrape sides. Add water, lemon juice and orange peel. Pulse twice; scrape sides. Pour into a 13x9x2-inch pan. Freeze until firm, about 2 to 3 hours.

Remove from freezer and let stand 15 minutes. Cut into 1-inch chunks. With machine running, gradually drop in chunks; process until thickly pureed, scraping sides occasionally. Serve immediately or spoon into tightly covered container and freeze until firm. Remove from freezer about 20 minutes before serving to soften for easier serving.

Wash strawberries just before using; then hull. If frozen strawberries are used, reduce freezer time from 2 to 3 hours to about 1 hour. Proceed as directed.

PEACHY NONFAT ICE CREAM

IF YOU OWN AN ICE CREAM MACHINE, THIS RECIPE IS FOR YOU
Prep time: 70 min   Freeze time: 2 hrs
Servings: 10   Serving size: 3/4 Cup
Exchanges: 1/2 Skim milk and 1 Fruit (2 Carbohydrate Choices)
Analysis per serving: 125 Calories, 24 g Carbohydrate, 6 g Protein,
1 g Fat, 2 mg Cholesterol, 96 mg Sodium, 1 g Fiber

2	**cups peaches, peeled and finely chopped (3-4 medium)**
1/4	**cup sugar**
1	**Tbs lemon juice**
2	**cups evaporated skim milk, chilled**
1	**cup skim milk**
1/2	**cup egg substitute**
1	**tsp dried lemon peel or grated fresh lemon peel**
1/2	**cup low-sugar raspberry jam**

In medium bowl, combine chopped peaches, sugar and lemon juice. Cover and refrigerate 1 hour, stirring frequently.

Shake evaporated milk and pour into medium bowl. Stir in skim milk, egg substitute and lemon peel; using electric mixer at medium speed, beat until well blended, scraping sides of bowl occasionally. Use a rubber spatula to stir in peach mixture and raspberry jam until well mixed.

Pour into freezer can of 1-gallon ice cream maker. Prepare ice cream according to manufacturer's instructions. Cover and freeze about 1 hour before serving.

❖ To peel peaches, plunge peaches into pot of boiling water and cook for 30 seconds; drain. Rinse with cold water; drain. Peel should slide off.

LIGHT & FRUITY SHAKE

SO GOOD, YOU WON'T BELIEVE IT'S FAT FREE
Prep time: 3 min   Cook time: 0 min
Servings: 2   Serving size: 1 Cup
Exchanges: 1/2 Skim Milk and 1 Fruit (1 Carbohydrate Choice)
Analysis per serving: 97 Calories, 20 g Carbohydrate, 5 g Protein,
0 g Fat, 2 mg Cholesterol, 63 mg Sodium, 1 g Fiber

1	cup skim milk
1	small ripe banana, thinly sliced
1	Tbs chocolate extract
4 or 5	ice cubes

In food processor, combine milk, sliced banana and extract. Whirl to
blend. Scrape sides. With machine running, add ice cubes one at a time,
and whirl until smooth. Serve immediately.

❖ 1 Tbs strawberry extract may be substituted.

FROZEN YOGURT POPS

A FAVORITE WITH KIDS OF ALL AGES
Prep time: 5 min   Cook time: 2 hrs
Serves: 6   Serving size: 1 Pop
Exchanges: 1/2 Skim Milk and 1 Fruit (2 Carbohydrate Choices)
Analysis per serving: 115 Calories, 25 g Carbohydrate, 4 g Protein,
0 g Fat, 0 mg Cholesterol, 45 mg Sodium, 0 Fiber

2	**cups plain nonfat yogurt**
1	**Tbs sugar**
1	**tsp vanilla extract**
2/3	**cup low-sugar strawberry jam**

Put all ingredients in a medium bowl and beat with electric mixer at medium speed or whirl in blender or process in food processor until frothy and well mixed, about 30 seconds.

Pour mixture into six 3-ounce paper cups and freeze about 1 hour. Insert wooden sticks into center of each cup and freeze until yogurt mixture is firm, about 1 hour. Peel paper cups from yogurt pops before eating.

TROPICAL AMBROSIA BARS

THESE BARS ARE NICE SERVED AT A LADIES LUNCHEON
Prep time: 10 min   Chill time: 2 hrs
Serves: 12   Serving size: 1 Bar, 1/12 Portion
Exchanges: 1/2 Fruit and 1 Fat (1 Carbohydrate Choice)
Analysis per serving: 69 Calories, 8 g Carbohydrate, 3 g Protein,
4 g Fat, 0 mg Cholesterol, 7 mg Sodium, 1 g Fiber

1	8-ounce can unsweetened, crushed pineapple
3	envelopes unflavored gelatin
1/2	cup chopped walnuts, toasted
1/2	cup raisins
1/4	cup flaked coconut

Strain pineapple, into a 4-cup measuring cup. Add enough water to measure 1 cup of liquid. Reserve crushed pineapple. Sprinkle gelatin over juice and water. Let sit 1 minute to soften. Stir and microwave on High for 3 minutes or until gelatin is dissolved. Let rest 1 minute.

Stir in reserved crushed pineapple and remaining ingredients. Mix well and turn into a 8 or 9-inch square pan. Chill about 2 hours or until firm. Cut into small squares.

HOMEMADE DRIED FRUIT

WHEN YOU MAKE YOUR OWN, THERE ARE NO PRESERVATIVES ADDED
Prep time: 20 min   Bake time: 4 hrs
Makes: 3 Cups   Serving size: 1/2 Cup, 1/6 Portion
Exchanges: 1 Fruit (1 Carbohydrate Choice)
Analysis per serving: 61 Calories, 16 g Carbohydrate, 0 g Protein,
0 g Fat, 0 mg Cholesterol, 2 mg Sodium, 2 g Fiber

4	**cups of water**
1/4	**cup lemon juice**
4	**large apples or pears**

Heat oven to 170°F or lowest temperature setting. Have baking sheets ready.

In a large bowl or salad spinner, mix water and lemon juice; set aside. Wash fruit, cut into quarters and remove seeds. Slice each quarter into 1/4-inch slices. Or, use slicing disc in food processor to slice thinly.

Drop fruit slices into water/lemon mixture and soak for 3 minutes. Drain and pat dry on paper towels or spin dry in salad spinner.

Arrange slices in a single layer on baking sheets. Place in oven on both oven racks. Leave door ajar about 1 inch. If necessary, prop door open with a wooden spoon. Let dry in oven 4 to 6 hours, rotating cookie sheets and turning slices over every 2 hours until slices are leathery and dry to the touch yet pliable.

Cool and store in tightly covered container or in plastic bags.

Muffins

Muffins are a treat any time of day. We usually associate muffins with breakfast, but they are luscious for lunch or dinner when served with a salad or soup. Muffins are terrific for a quick and healthy snack since they are filling and have a touch of sweetness.

When you are short on time but want a homemade snack, whip up a batch of muffins. They are quick and simple to make with very little fuss. There is no need to take out the electric mixer. You can also assemble and mix the dry ingredients in one bowl and mix the wet ingredients in another bowl ahead of time. When ready to bake, combine dry and wet ingredients and promptly bake, unless recipe states otherwise.

As you can see from the following recipes, I have used whole-wheat flour in just about every recipe. Whole-wheat flour adds fiber which is a necessary diet staple. If you prefer lighter muffins, simply use only all-purpose flour instead of a mixture of whole-wheat and all-purpose flours.

Some of my muffin recipes call for old-fashioned oatmeal which has more fiber than quick-cooking oatmeal. I prefer using the more fibrous oatmeal. Use whichever one you prefer.

These muffin recipes are low in sugar. I do not use artificial sweeteners. Instead, I use a minimum amount of sugar and fruit or fruit juice for added sweetness.

Here are a few suggestions for delicious muffins. Read the recipe before attempting to mix muffins. Have all ingredients and equipment ready so that you don't waste time searching for items necessary to prepare the recipe. Follow directions carefully. Before spooning batter into prepared muffin tins, read over the recipe again just in case you overlooked an ingredient.

Muffins should not be overmixed because it will make them tough. Liquid ingredients should be added to dry ingredients and mixed just enough to dampen all the flour. The batter should be rough and lumpy. When adding nuts or fruit, mix them with the flour before adding the liquids to avoid extra stirring.

Knobs, peaks or tunnels in your muffins are caused by over mixing or oven temperatures that are too low or too high. Spoon batter into muffin tins which have been sprayed with cooking spray or lined with cupcake paper liners. When filling prepared muffin tins, fill about two-thirds full. Too much batter in muffin tins will cause the muffins to spill over. Too little batter in the muffin tins will result in flat, short muffins.

Unless the recipe specifies, muffins should be removed from baking tins immediately and served or put on racks to cool. When cool, store covered at room temperature or freeze up to 3 months. Many of my muffin recipes contain fruit for added sweetness; therefore, they cannot remain at room temperature for more than 2 days. Fruit added to baked items makes them moister, sweeter and more flavorful. But, if left at room temperature too long, they will spoil. Refrigeration helps retain freshness. Just reheat in microwave or toaster oven before serving.

To defrost frozen muffins, leave at room temperature for about an hour or place on a paper towel or paper plate and defrost on High in the microwave for 1 minute. You might want to microwave another 40 seconds if you prefer to eat it immediately. Or, defrost then split and toast until warm. For variety, mini muffins can be made using mini muffin tins. Muffins are a joy to bake and are so simple to make.

APPETIZING APPLE MUFFINS

THE SECRET INGREDIENT IS MAPLE EXTRACT
Prep time: 10 min   Bake time: 20 min
Makes: 12   Serving size: 1 Muffin
Exchanges: 1 Starch and 1/2 Fat (1 Carbohydrate Choice)
Analysis per serving: 109 Calories, 16 g Carbohydrate, 3 g Protein,
4 g Fat, 0 mg Cholesterol, 170 mg Sodium, 2 Fiber

3/4	cup whole-wheat flour
1/2	cup all-purpose flour
1	cup old-fashioned oats
3	Tbs brown sugar
1	Tbs baking powder
1/4	tsp salt
1	tsp cinnamon
1/4	tsp nutmeg
1	cup apple, peeled, cored & chopped (1 medium)
2	large egg whites or 1/4 cup egg substitute
3	Tbs olive or canola oil
1	cup skim milk
1	tsp maple extract

Preheat oven 400°F. Spray 12 muffin baking tins with cooking spray or line with paper liners.

In a large bowl, combine flours, oatmeal, sugar, baking powder, salt and spices; stir in chopped apple until coated with flour mixture.

In a small bowl, use a whisk or a fork to combine egg whites, oil, milk and extract. Stir blended wet ingredients into flour mixture. Blend until flour is moistened; do not overmix.

Spoon batter into prepared muffin tins. Bake 20 to 25 minutes or until browned and pick inserted in center comes out clean. Immediately remove from tins. Serve or cool on rack. Store covered and/or freeze.

APPLE SPICE MUFFINS

STORE THESE MUFFINS OVERNIGHT TO DEVELOP THE FLAVOR
Prep time: 10 min   Bake time: 20 min
Makes: 12   Serving size: 1 Muffin
Exchanges: 1/2 Starch, 1/2 Fruit and 1/2 Fat (1 Carbohydrate Choice)
Analysis per serving: 112 Calories, 19 g Carbohydrate, 3 g Protein,
3 g Fat, 0 mg Cholesterol, 162 mg Sodium, 2 g Fiber

3/4	cup all-purpose flour
1/2	cup whole-wheat flour
3/4	cup old-fashioned oats
1	Tbs baking powder
1/2	tsp cinnamon
1/4	tsp ginger
1/4	tsp salt
2	Tbs sugar
1	medium apple, unpeeled, finely chopped
3	Tbs raisins
2	large egg whites or 1/4 cup egg substitute
3/4	cup skim milk
2	Tbs olive or canola oil
1	tsp vanilla

Preheat oven 400°F. Spray 12 muffin tins with cooking spray or line with muffin papers.

In a large bowl, combine flours, oats, baking powder, cinnamon, ginger, salt and sugar until blended. Stir in chopped apple and raisins until fruit is coated with flour mixture.

In a small bowl, use a whisk or a fork to combine egg whites, milk, oil and vanilla. Add wet ingredients to dry ingredients and mix just until blended; do not overmix.

Spoon into prepared muffin tins. Bake 20 minutes or until browned and when pick inserted in center of muffin comes out clean. Immediately remove baked muffins from tins. Cool on rack. Store covered and/or freeze.

BANANA POPPY SEED MUFFINS

1	cup whole-wheat flour
1	cup all-purpose flour
2	Tbs sugar
1	Tbs baking powder
1/8	tsp salt
2	Tbs poppy seeds
1/2	cup mashed ripe banana (1 medium)
1	tsp dried lemon peel or grated fresh lemon peel
3	Tbs olive or canola oil
2	large egg whites or 1/4 cup egg substitute
1	cup buttermilk

Preheat oven 400°F. Spray 12 muffin baking tins with cooking spray or line with muffin papers.

In large bowl, combine flours, sugar, baking powder, salt and poppy seeds.

In small bowl, use a whisk or a fork to combine mashed banana, lemon peel, oil, egg whites and buttermilk until well blended. Add wet ingredients to dry ingredients and stir just until blended; do not overmix.

Spoon batter into prepared pans. Bake 20 minutes or until pick inserted in center comes out clean. Immediately remove from tins. Serve or place on rack to cool completely. Store covered and/or freeze.

BLUEBERRY MUFFINS

A MUFFIN LOVERS FAVORITE MUFFIN
Prep time: 10 min   Bake time: 20 min
Makes: 12   Serving size: 1 Muffin
Exchanges: 1 Starch, 1 Fruit and 1/2 Fat (1 Carbohydrate Choice)
Analysis per serving: 131 Calories, 21 g Carbohydrate, 4 g Protein,
4 g Fat, 1mg Cholesterol, 181 mg Sodium, 2 g Fiber

1	cup whole-wheat flour
1	cup all-purpose flour
3	Tbs sugar
1	Tbs baking powder
1/2	tsp nutmeg
1/4	tsp salt
1	cup fresh or frozen blueberries
2	large egg whites or 1/4 cup egg substitute
1	cup buttermilk
3	Tbs olive or canola oil
1	tsp dried lemon peel or grated fresh lemon peel

Preheat oven 400°F. Spray 12 muffin baking tins with cooking spray or line with paper liners.

In a large bowl, combine flours, sugar, baking powder and spices. Gently stir in blueberries until blueberries are coated with flour mixture.

In a small bowl, use a whisk or a fork to combine egg whites, buttermilk, olive oil and lemon peel. Add to blueberry mixture and stir just until blended; do not overmix.

Spoon batter into prepared pans. Bake 20 to 25 minutes or until browned and pick inserted in center comes out clean. Immediately remove from baking tins and cool on rack. Serve warm. Store covered and/or freeze.

CHOCOLATE CHIP MUFFINS

YOU WON'T BELIEVE THEIR GREAT TASTE
Prep time: 10 min   Bake time: 15 min
Makes:12   Serving size: 1 Muffin
Exchanges: 1 1/2 Starch and 1 Fat (2 Carbohydrate Choices)
Analysis per serving: 160 Calories, 24 g Carbohydrate, 3 g Protein,
6 g Fat, 0 mg Cholesterol, 165 mg Sodium, 2 g Fiber

1	cup whole-wheat flour
1	cup all-purpose flour
1	Tbs baking powder
1/4	tsp salt
1	Tbs brown sugar
1	Tbs sugar
1/3	cup mini chocolate chips
2	large egg whites or 1/4 cup egg substitute
3	Tbs olive or canola oil
1/2	cup orange juice
1/2	cup skim milk
1/2	tsp vanilla extract
1/2	tsp butter extract (optional)

Preheat oven 400°F. Spray 12 muffin tins with cooking spray or line with paper liners.

In medium bowl, combine flours, baking powder, salt, sugars and chips. In a small bowl, use a whisk or a fork to combine egg whites, oil, juice, milk; vanilla extract and butter extract (if using).

Add wet ingredients to dry ingredients and combine just until moistened. Do not overmix.

Spoon into prepared muffin tins. Bake 15 to 20 minutes until browned and pick inserted in center comes out clean. Immediately remove from baking tins. Serve or cool on rack. Store covered or freeze.

CORN MUFFINS

GREAT FOR BREAKFAST OR A TASTY ADDITION TO LUNCH OR DINNER
Prep time: 10 min   Bake time: 20 min
Makes: 12   Serving size: 1 Muffin
Exchanges: 1 Starch and 1/2 Fat (1 Carbohydrate Choice)
Analysis per serving: 126 Calories, 20 g Carbohydrate, 3 g Protein,
4 g Fat, 0 mg Cholesterol, 170 mg Sodium, 2 g Fiber

1	**cup corn meal**
1/2	**cup whole-wheat flour**
1/2	**cup all-purpose flour**
2	**Tbs sugar**
1	**Tbs baking powder**
1/4	**tsp salt**
3	**Tbs olive or canola oil**
1	**Tbs butter extract**
1	**cup skim milk or buttermilk**
2	**large egg whites or 1/4 cup egg substitute**

Preheat oven 425°F. Spray 12 muffin tins with cooking spray or line with paper muffin liners.

In a large bowl, combine corn meal, flours, sugar, baking powder and salt.

In a small bowl, using a whisk or a fork, mix oil, butter extract, milk and egg whites until well blended. Stir wet ingredients into dry ingredients until mixture is moistened; do not overmix. Spoon into prepared muffin tins.

Bake 20 minutes or until browned and pick inserted in center comes out clean. Immediately remove from tins. Serve or place on rack to cool completely. Store covered and/or freeze.

CORNBREAD: Prepare as directed above and pour into a 9x9x2-inch pan which has been sprayed with cooking spray. Bake 20 or 25 minutes or until browned and pick inserted in center comes out clean. Cut into squares and serve warm.

BLUEBERRY CORN MUFFINS

A DIFFERENT TASTE TO CORN MUFFINS — SPECTACULAR!
Prep time: 10 min   Bake time: 20 min
Makes: 12   Serving size: 1 Muffin
Exchanges: 1 Starch, 1/2 Fruit and 1/2 Fat (1 Carbohydrate Choice)
Analysis per serving: 134 Calories, 22 g Carbohydrate, 4 g Protein,
4 g Fat, 0 mg Cholesterol, 170 mg Sodium, 2 g Fiber

Prepare CORN MUFFIN recipe on preceding page as directed and add
the following ingredients to the dry ingredients.

  1   cup fresh or frozen blueberries
  1/4   tsp nutmeg
  1/2   tsp dried lemon peel or grated fresh lemon peel

Proceed as directed.

CRANBERRY MUFFINS

THESE MUFFINS TASTE JUST LIKE CRANBERRY BREAD
Prep time: 10 min   Bake time: 15 min
Makes: 12   Serving size: 1 Muffin
Exchanges: 1/2 Starch, 1/2 Fruit and 1/2 Fat (1 Carbohydrate Choice)
Analysis per serving: 114 Calories, 18 g Carbohydrate, 3 g Protein,
4 g Fat, 0 mg Cholesterol, 205 mg Sodium, 2 g Fiber

1/4	**cup chopped nuts (optional)**
3/4	**cup whole-wheat flour**
3/4	**cup all-purpose flour**
3	**Tbs sugar**
1	**Tbs baking powder**
1/2	**tsp baking soda**
1/4	**tsp salt**
1/4	**tsp nutmeg**
1	**Tbs dried orange peel or grated fresh orange peel**
1	**cup cranberries, washed & drained (fresh or frozen)**
2	**large egg whites or 1/4 cup egg substitute**
3	**Tbs olive or canola oil**
1	**cup orange juice**

Preheat oven 400°F. If using nuts, place on baking sheet and bake 3 to 5 minutes or until toasted; set aside. Spray 12 muffin tins with cooking spray or line with paper muffin liners.

Sift flours, sugar, baking powder, soda and orange peel into a large bowl. Stir in toasted nuts (if using) and cranberries until mixed.

In a small bowl, use a whisk or a fork to combine egg whites, oil and orange juice. Add wet ingredients to dry ingredients and stir just until moistened. Do not overmix.

Spoon batter into prepared muffin tins. Bake 15 to 18 minutes or until golden brown and pick inserted in center comes out clean. Immediately remove from tins. Serve or cool on rack completely. Store covered and/or freeze.

FRUITY BRAN MUFFINS

FRUIT JUICE & DRIED FRUIT ADD FLAVOR & NATURAL SWEETNESS
Prep time: 10 min   Bake time: 20 min
Makes: 12   Serving size: 1 Muffin
Exchanges: 1/2 Starch, 1/2 Fruit and 1/2 Fat (1 Carbohydrate Choice)
Analysis per serving: 117 Calories, 20 g Carbohydrate, 3 g Protein,
4 g Fat, 0 mg Cholesterol, 111 mg Sodium, 3 g Fiber

1	cup wheat bran
1	cup unsweetened fruit juice (your choice)
1/2	cup whole-wheat flour
1/2	cup all-purpose flour
1/4	cup old-fashioned oats
1	Tbs sugar
1	Tbs baking powder
1/2	tsp cinnamon
1/4	tsp nutmeg
3	Tbs raisins or chopped dates
2	large egg whites or 1/4 cup egg substitute
3	Tbs olive or canola oil
1/2	cup mashed banana (1 medium)

Preheat oven 400°F. Spray 12 muffin tins with cooking spray or line with
paper baking cups.

In a small bowl, stir wheat bran into fruit juice; let rest 5 minutes to soften.

In a large bowl, combine flours, oatmeal, sugar, baking powder and
spices. Stir in raisins or chopped dates and the bran/fruit juice mixture.

In bowl used to combine bran and juice, use a whisk or a fork to beat egg
whites and olive oil; stir in mashed banana. Add wet ingredients to flour
mixture. Combine just until moistened; do not overmix.

Spoon batter into prepared baking tins. Bake 20 to 25 minutes or until
golden brown or pick inserted in center comes out clean. Immediately
remove from baking tins. Serve or cool on rack. Store covered.

HONEY BRAN MUFFINS

A DELICIOUS HEALTHY MUFFIN
Prep time: 10 min   Bake time: 18 min
Makes:12   Serving size: 1 Muffin
Exchanges: 1/2 Starch, 1/2 Fruit and 1 Fat (1 Carbohydrate Choice)
Analysis per serving: 130 Calories, 21 g Carbohydrate, 4 g Protein,
5 g Fat, 0 mg Cholesterol, 136 mg Sodium, 4 g Fiber

1 1/4	**cups wheat bran**
3/4	**cup all-purpose flour**
1/2	**cup whole-wheat flour**
2	**tsp baking powder**
1/4	**tsp salt**
1/4	**cup olive or canola oil**
1/4	**cup honey**
1	**cup skim milk**
2	**large egg whites**

Preheat oven 375°F. Spray 12 muffin tins with cooking spray or line with paper liners.

In a large bowl, combine bran, flours, baking powder and salt.

In small bowl, using a whisk or fork, combine oil, honey, milk and egg whites until well blended. Add wet ingredients to dry ingredients and mix just until blended; do not overmix.

Spoon into prepared muffin tins and bake 18 to 24 minutes or until browned and pick inserted into center of muffin comes out clean. Immediately remove baked muffins from tin. Serve or cool completely on rack. Store covered and/or freeze.

ISLAND MUFFINS

ORANGE AND PINEAPPLE GIVE THESE MUFFINS A TROPICAL TASTE
Prep time: 10 min   Bake time: 15 min
Makes : 12   Serving size: 1 Muffin
Exchanges: 1 Starch, 1/2 Fruit and 1/2 Fat (1 Carbohydrate Choice)
Analysis per serving: 131 Calories, 22 g Carbohydrate, 3 g Protein,
3 g Fat, 0 mg Cholesterol, 164 mg Sodium, 2 g Fiber

1	cup whole-wheat flour
1	cup all-purpose flour
1	Tbs baking powder
1/4	tsp salt
3	Tbs sugar
2	large egg whites or 1/4 cup egg substitute
3	Tbs olive or canola oil
2	tsp dried orange peel or grated fresh orange peel
1/2	cup orange juice
1	8-ounce can juice-packed crushed pineapple, undrained

Preheat oven 400°F. Spray 12 muffin tins with cooking spray or line with paper baking cups.

In medium bowl, combine flours, baking powder, salt and sugar; set aside.

In small bowl, use a whisk or a fork to combine egg whites, oil, orange peel, orange juice and undrained crushed pineapple. Stir into dry ingredients just until moistened; do not overmix.

Spoon in prepared muffin tins. Bake 15 to 18 minutes or until golden brown and pick inserted in center comes out clean. Immediately remove from baking tins and serve. Cool completely on rack. Store covered and/or freeze.

LUSCIOUS
RASPBERRY MUFFINS

DON'T WAIT FOR SUMMER TO ENJOY THESE MUFFINS
Prep time: 10 min `   Bake time: 15 min
Makes: 12   Serving size: 1 Muffin
Exchanges: 1 Starch, 1/2 Fruit and 1/2 Fat (2 Carbohydrate Choices)
Analysis per serving: 148 Calories, 24 g Carbohydrate, 5 g Protein,
4 g Fat, 1 mg Cholesterol, 190 mg Sodium, 2 g Fiber

1/4	cup chopped nuts (optional)
1	cup whole-wheat flour
1	cup all-purpose flour
1/4	cup nonfat dry milk powder
3	Tbs sugar
1	Tbs baking powder
1/2	tsp baking soda
2	cups frozen or fresh raspberries (washed & drained)
1/4	cup bran flakes
2	large egg whites or 1/4 cup egg substitute
3	Tbs olive or canola oil
1	cup orange juice
2	tsp dried orange peel or grated fresh orange peel

Preheat oven 400°F. Spray 12 muffin tins with cooking spray or line with paper baking cups. If using nuts, place on baking sheet and bake 3 to 5 minutes or until toasted; set aside.

Sift flours, dry milk, sugar, baking powder and baking soda into a medium bowl. If grains remain in sifter, stir into dry ingredients. Use a rubber spatula to gently stir raspberries, bran flakes and toasted nuts (if using) into dry ingredients.

In a small bowl, use a whisk or a fork to combine egg whites, oil, juice and orange peel until well mixed. Use a rubber spatula to gently stir blended liquids into raspberry mixture; combine just until moistened. Do not overmix.

Spoon batter into prepared muffin tins. Bake 15 to 18 minutes or until golden brown and pick inserted in center comes out clean. Immediately remove from tins. Serve or place on rack to cool completely. Store covered and/or freeze.

MAPLE NUT MUFFINS

MARVELOUS MUFFINS
Prep time: 10 min   Bake time: 20 min
Makes: 12   Serving size: 1 Muffin
Exchanges: 1 Starch and 1 Fat (1 Carbohydrate Choice)
Analysis per serving: 137 Calories, 20 g Carbohydrate, 4 g Protein,
5 g Fat, 0 mg Cholesterol, 121 mg Sodium, 2 g Fiber

1/4	cup chopped pecans
1	cup whole-wheat flour
1	cup all-purpose flour
1	Tbs baking powder
1/4	cup low-calorie maple syrup
2	large egg whites or 1/4 cup egg substitute
1	cup skim milk
2	tsp maple extract
3	Tbs olive or canola oil

Preheat oven 400°F. Put nuts on baking sheet and bake for 3 to 5 minutes or until lightly toasted; set aside.

Spray 12 muffin tins with cooking spray or line with paper baking cups.

In medium mixing bowl, combine flours and baking powder; stir in toasted nuts. In small bowl, use a whisk or a fork to combine syrup, egg whites, milk, extract and oil until well blended. Pour blended liquid ingredients into dry ingredients; stir just until moistened Do not overmix.

Spoon into prepared baking tins. Bake 20 to 25 minutes or until golden brown and pick inserted in center comes out clean. Remove immediately. Serve or cool completely on rack. Store covered and/or freeze.

PEANUT BUTTER
& JELLY MUFFINS

A FAVORITE SANDWICH IN A MUFFIN
Prep time: 10 min   Bake time: 15 min
Makes: 12   Serving size: 1 Muffin
Exchanges:1/2 Lean meat, 1 Starch, 1/2 Fruit and 1 1/2 Fat (2 Carbohydrate Choices)
Analysis per serving: 202 Calories, 24 g Carbohydrate, 7 g Protein,
9 g Fat, 0 mg Cholesterol, 179 mg Sodium, 2 g Fiber

1/2	cup yellow cornmeal
1/2	cup whole-wheat flour
1	cup all-purpose flour
1	Tbs brown sugar
1	Tbs sugar
1/4	tsp salt
1	Tbs baking powder
3	large egg whites
3	Tbs olive or canola oil
1/2	cup natural peanut butter
1	cup skim milk
1/2	cup orange juice
2	Tbs low-sugar jelly or jam of your choice

Preheat oven 425°F. Spray 12 muffin tins with cooking spray or line with paper baking cups.

Sift cornmeal, flours, sugars, salt and baking powder into a medium bowl; set aside.

In a small bowl, use a whisk or a fork to combine egg whites, oil, peanut butter, milk and orange juice until well blended. Add liquid ingredients to dry ingredients; stir with a rubber spatula just until moistened; do not over mix.

Spoon batter into prepared baking tins. Drop about 1/2 teaspoon of jam or jelly in center of each muffin; pressing jam or jelly in slightly. Bake 15 to 20 minutes or until golden brown and pick inserted in center, comes out clean. Immediately remove from baking tins. Serve or cool on racks. Store covered and/or freeze.

POPULAR POPPY SEED MUFFINS

ABSOLUTELY SCRUMPTIOUS
Prep time: 10 min   Bake time: 20 min
Makes: 12   Serving size:1 Muffin
Exchanges: 1 Starch, 1/2 Fruit and 1 1/2 Fat (2 Carbohydrate Choices)
Analysis per serving: 168 Calories, 23 g Carbohydrate, 4 g Protein,
7 g Fat, 18 mg Cholesterol, 154 mg Sodium, 2 g Fiber

1/4	cup chopped pecans
1	cup all-purpose flour
1	cup whole-wheat flour
3	Tbs sugar
2 1/2	tsp baking powder
1/4	tsp salt
1/4	tsp nutmeg
1/4	cup golden raisins
5	Tbs poppy seeds
1/4	cup olive or canola oil
1	large egg
2	large egg whites or 1/4 cup egg substitute
1/2	tsp dried orange peel or grated fresh lemon peel
1/2	cup orange juice
1/2	cup skim milk

Preheat oven 400°F. Spray 12 muffin tins with cooking spray or line with paper liners. Place nuts on baking sheet and bake 3 to 5 minutes or until toasted.

In a large bowl, combine flours, sugar, baking powder, salt, nutmeg, raisins, poppy seeds and toasted pecans; set aside.

In a small bowl, use a whisk or a fork to combine oil, egg, egg whites, orange peel, juice and milk. Add wet ingredients to dry ingredients and mix just until blended; do not overmix.

Spoon into muffin tins and bake for about 20 minutes or until pick inserted in center comes out clean. Immediately remove from tins. Serve or place on rack to cool completely. Store covered and/or freeze up to 3 months.

PUMPKIN MUFFINS

A PERFECT SUBSTITUTE FOR PUMPKIN BREAD
Prep time: 10 min   Bake time: 20 min
Makes: 12   Serving size: 1 Muffin
Exchanges: 1/2 Starch, 1/2 Fruit and 1 Fat (1 Carbohydrate Choice)
Analysis per serving: 147 Calories, 19 g Carbohydrate, 4 g Protein,
7 g Fat, 0 mg Cholesterol, 221 mg Sodium, 2 g Fiber

1/4	cup chopped pecans
3/4	cup whole-wheat flour
1/2	cup all-purpose flour
1/2	cup wheat germ
1	tsp baking soda
2	tsp baking powder
1/4	tsp salt
1/2	tsp cinnamon
1/4	tsp nutmeg
2	large egg whites or 1/4 cup egg substitute
1/4	cup olive or canola oil
1	cup pureed cooked pumpkin or canned pumpkin (NOT pie filling)
2	Tbs honey
2	Tbs molasses
1/4	cup orange juice

Preheat oven 375°F. Place nuts on baking sheet and bake for 3 to 5 minutes or until toasted; set aside. Spray 12 muffin tins with cooking spray or line with paper muffin liners.

In a large bowl, combine flours, wheat germ, baking soda, baking powder, salt and spices; stir in toasted nuts. Set aside.

In small bowl, use a whisk or a fork to combine egg whites, oil, pumpkin, honey, molasses and orange juice. Add blended wet ingredients to flour mixture. Combine just until blended; do not overmix.

Spoon mixture in prepared muffin tins. Bake 20 minutes or until lightly browned and pick inserted in center comes out clean. Cool muffins in tins on rack for 5 minutes. Then, remove muffins. Serve warm or cool completely on rack. Store covered and/or freeze.

RASPBERRY
SURPRISE MUFFINS

A SWEET SURPRISE IN THE MUFFIN MIDDLE
Prep time: 15 min   Bake time: 20 min
Makes:12   Serving size: 1 Muffin
Exchanges: 1/2 Starch, 1/2 Fruit and 1 Fat (1 Carbohydrate Choice)
Analysis per serving: 130 Calories, 19 g Carbohydrate, 3 g Protein,
5 g Fat, 0 mg Cholesterol, 154 mg Sodium, 1 g Fiber

3/4	cup whole-wheat flour
3/4	cup all-purpose flour
2 1/2	tsp baking powder
1/4	tsp salt
1	tsp cinnamon
2 1/2	Tbs nonfat dry milk powder or buttermilk powder
1/4	cup sugar
2	large egg whites
3/4	cup orange juice
1/4	cup olive or canola oil
3	Tbs low-sugar raspberry jam or preserves

Preheat oven 400°F. Spray 12 muffin tins with cooking spray or line with
paper liners.

In a large bowl, combine flours, baking powder, salt, cinnamon, dry milk
and sugar. Make a well in center of mixture. Set aside.

In a small bowl, use a whisk or a fork to combine egg whites, juice and oil.
Pour into flour well and mix just until blended. Do not overmix.

Spoon one heaping tablespoon of batter into prepared muffin tins. Drop
about 1/2 teaspoon of raspberry jam or preserves into center of each
muffin; do not spread. Top with another tablespoon of batter onto each
muffin.

Bake 20 minutes or until golden brown and tops spring back when
touched lightly in center. Immediately remove muffins from tins. Serve or
cool on rack. When cool, store covered or freeze up to 3 months.

SCRUMPTIOUS
STRAWBERRY MUFFINS

IT'S HARD TO EAT JUST ONE
Prep time: 10 min   Bake time: 20 min
Makes: 12   Serving size: 1 Muffin
Exchanges: 1 Starch, 1/2 Fruit and 1/2 Fat (1 Carbohydrate Choice)
Analysis per serving: 126 Calories, 22 g Carbohydrate, 4 g Protein,
3 g Fat, 1 mg Cholesterol, 132 mg Sodium, 2 g Fiber

1	cup all-purpose flour
1	cup whole-wheat flour
3	Tbs sugar
1	Tbs baking powder
1/2	tsp cinnamon
1	cup coarsely chopped fresh or slightly thawed frozen strawberries
2	large egg whites or 1/4 cup egg substitute
2	Tbs olive or canola oil
1	cup buttermilk
2	Tbs orange juice
1/2	tsp vanilla extract
1	tsp dried orange peel or grated fresh orange peel

Preheat oven 400°F. Spray 12 muffin tins with cooking spray or line with paper muffin liners. Sift flours, sugar, baking powder and cinnamon into a large bowl. If grains remain in sifter, stir into dry ingredients. Stir in chopped strawberries and coat with flour mixture.

In a small bowl, use a whisk or a fork to combine egg whites, oil, buttermilk, orange juice, extract and peel. Add blended liquids to flour mixture. Mix until dry ingredients are just moistened; do not overmix.

Spoon batter into prepared muffin tins. Bake 20 minutes or until lightly brown and pick inserted in center comes out clean. Immediately remove from muffin tins. Serve or cool on rack. Store covered and/or freeze.

SPICY GINGER MUFFINS

IF YOU LOVE GINGERBREAD, YOU'LL ENJOY EVERY BITE
Prep time: 10 min   Bake time: 20 min
Makes: 12   Serving size: 1 Muffin
Exchanges: 1 Starch, 1/2 Fruit and 1/2 Fat (1 Carbohydrate Choice)
Analysis per serving: 132 Calories, 21 g Carbohydrate, 4 g Protein,
4 g Fat, 1 mg Cholesterol, 163 mg Sodium, 2 g Fiber

1	cup whole-wheat flour
1	cup all-purpose flour
1	Tbs brown sugar
2	tsp ground ginger
1	tsp cinnamon
1/4	tsp cloves
1	Tbs baking powder
1/8	tsp salt
1	cup buttermilk
2	large egg whites or 1/4 cup egg substitute
2	Tbs orange juice
1/2	tsp vanilla extract
3	Tbs olive or canola oil
1/4	cup molasses

Preheat oven 400°F. Spray 12 muffin tins with cooking spray or line with
paper muffin liners.   In a large bowl, combine flours, sugar, spices, baking
powder and salt; set aside.

In a small bowl, use a whisk or a fork to combine buttermilk, egg whites,
juice, extract, oil and molasses until well blended.   Form a well in center
of flour mixture. Pour in wet ingredients and stir just until moistened. Do
not overmix.

Spoon batter into prepared muffin tins and bake 20 to 25 minutes or until
browned and pick inserted in center comes out clean. Immediately
remove from baking tins and serve.   Or, cool on rack. Store covered
and/or freeze.

ZANY ZUCCHINI MUFFINS

GREAT FOR BREAKFAST, LUNCH, DINNER OR A SNACK
Prep time: 10 min   Bake time: 20 min
Makes: 12   Serving size: 1 Muffin
Exchanges: 1 Starch, 1/2 Fruit and 1/2 Fat (1 Carbohydrate Choice)
Analysis per serving: 128 Calories, 21 g Carbohydrate, 4 g Protein,
4 g Fat, 0 mg Cholesterol, 167 mg Sodium, 2 g Fiber

1	cup whole-wheat flour
1	cup all-purpose flour
1	Tbs baking powder
1/4	tsp salt
1/4	cup sugar
1	tsp dried lemon peel or grated fresh lemon peel
1/4	tsp nutmeg
1	cup shredded zucchini
3/4	cup skim milk
3	Tbs olive or canola oil
2	large egg whites or 1/4 cup egg substitute

Preheat oven 400°F. Spray 12 muffin tins with cooking spray or line with paper liners.

In a large bowl, combine flours, baking powder, salt, sugar, peel and nutmeg. Make well in center of mixture; set aside.

In a small bowl, use a fork or a whisk to combine zucchini, milk, oil and egg whites until well blended. Add to flour mixture well and stir just until blended. Do not overmix.

Spoon into prepared tins and bake for 20 minutes or until golden brown. Immediately remove from tins. Serve or place on rack to cool completely. Store covered and/or freeze up to 3 months.

Pies

Everyone likes the smell of a pie baking. But they seem time-consuming and too hard to make. Most people reserve them for holidays and special occasions. It is possible to make delicious pies — cheaper and healthier than buying one at the store.

The recipes in this section are designed to be easier. Most of the crusts take less than 25 minutes from start to finish, and that includes baking! These recipes use only small amounts of sugar. Other ingredients help reduce fat, like nonfat yogurt, skim milk and nonfat ricotta cheese. Seasonal fruits, like fresh berries, add color, great taste and fiber.

This section also includes a few tart and cobbler recipes. Cobblers generally have a top crust but not one on the bottom. They are filled with fruit. Tarts are like pies with no top crust. Their fillings are jam or custard-like. Tart crusts are similar to a pastry crust, made with a little sugar and light butter. Pie crusts are often made with oil or shortening.

Look for the tasty, revised version of the traditional Greek pastry, Baklava. Traditionally made from layering clarified butter and a sugar syrup with phyllo (pronounced *filo*) pastry, the DIABETIC GOODIE BOOK Baklava is made by brushing a mixture of light butter/oil and a fruit syrup between phyllo layers. The nutrition comparison is staggering:

Traditional Baklava	*DIABETIC GOODIE BOOK* Baklava
226 Calories	38 Calories
22 g Carbohydrate	4 g Carbohydrate
15 g Fat	2 g Fat

CREAMY APPLE PIE
FILLING

PLAIN NONFAT YOGURT GIVES THIS PIE ITS CREAMINESS
Prep time: 10 min   Bake time: 35 min
Serves: 8   Serving size: 1 Slice, 1/8 Portion
Exchanges: 1/2 Starch and 1 Fruit (1 Carbohydrate Choice)
Analysis per serving: 98 Calories, 20 g Carbohydrate, 5 g Protein,
0 g Fat, 1 mg Cholesterol, 132 mg Sodium, 2 g Fiber (without crust)

3/4	cup egg substitute
2	Tbs all-purpose flour
1/4	tsp salt
1/2	tsp cinnamon
1/8	tsp nutmeg
1	cup plain nonfat yogurt
1/4	cup apple juice
1/4	tsp almond extract
3	cups peeled, cored & diced Golden Delicious apples (3 medium)
1/2	cup raisins (preferably white)
1	ZIP ZAP PIE CRUST (page 184) or OATMEAL CRUST (page 181), baked

Preheat oven to 350°F.

In medium bowl, use a whisk to beat egg substitute until frothy. On waxed paper or in small bowl, combine flour, salt and spices; add to beaten egg substitute, whisking until well blended; scrape sides of bowl. Whisk in yogurt, apple juice and almond extract until well mixed.

In medium bowl, combine apples and raisins; place in baked pie shell of your choice. Place pie shell on baking sheet to prevent spillovers. Pour egg mixture over apple mixture. Bake 35 to 40 minutes or until knife inserted in center comes out clean. Cool on rack 1 hour before serving. Cover and refrigerate leftovers.

POACHED STREUSEL APPLE PIE

BAKING TIME IS SHORTENED SINCE THE APPLES ARE PRECOOKED
Prep time: 20 min   Bake time: 20 min
Serves: 8   Serving size: 1 Slice, 1/8 Portion
Exchanges: 1 Starch, 2 Fruit and 2 Fat (3 Carbohydrate Choices)
Analysis per serving: 280 Calories, 48 g Carbohydrate, 3 g Protein,
10 g Fat, 0 mg Cholesterol, 136 mg Sodium, 3 g Fiber (with crust)

4	cups peeled, sliced apples (3-4 medium)
2	Tbs frozen concentrated apple juice, thawed
2	Tbs lemon juice & enough water to measure 1/3 cup
1	tsp cinnamon
1	tsp dried lemon peel or grated fresh lemon peel
1/4	cup white raisins
1	EASY PIE CRUST (page 182), baked
1	Tbs cornstarch
1	tsp water

Preheat oven to 350°F.

In large frying pan, combine apples, concentrated apple juice, lemon water, cinnamon, peel and raisins; bring to boil. Reduce heat and simmer 10 minutes. With slotted spoon, transfer apple mixture into baked pie crust. Combine cornstarch and water to make a thin paste. Add to liquid remaining in pan, cook and stir until thick; pour over apples. Sprinkle with streusel.

Streusel

1/4	cup whole-wheat flour
1/4	cup old-fashioned oats
1	tsp cinnamon
1/2	tsp nutmeg
1/4	cup chopped nuts
1	Tbs brown sugar
3	Tbs light margarine or light butter, thinly sliced

In medium bowl, combine flour, oats, spices, nuts and brown sugar. Using fork, pastry blender or two knives scissor-fashion, incorporate margarine until crumbly. Sprinkle over pie. Bake 20 to 25 minutes or until browned. If crust browns too much, cover edges with aluminum foil Serve warm. Cover and refrigerate leftovers.

❖ Try Rome Beauty, Granny Smith, Golden Delicious or Newtown Pippin apples.

COMPANY APPLE TART

COMPLIMENTS ARE FORTHCOMING WHEN THIS TART IS SERVED
Prep time: 10 min   Bake time: 40 min
Serves: 10   Serving size: 1 Slice, 1/10 Portion
Exchanges: 1 Starch, 1/2 Fruit and 1 Fat (2 Carbohydrate Choices)
Analysis per serving: 178 Calories, 24 g Carbohydrate, 6 Protein,
7 g Fat, 1 mg Cholesterol, 60 mg Sodium, 2 Fiber

3	apples, peeled, cored & cut into wedges
1/4	cup olive or canola oil
1	cup egg substitute
1	cup skim milk
1/4	cup plain nonfat yogurt
1/4	cup sugar
1/4	tsp nutmeg
1/2	tsp cinnamon
1	tsp lemon juice
1	Tbs vanilla extract
2	tsp almond extract
3/4	cup all-purpose flour
1/2	cup whole-wheat flour
2	Tbs sliced almonds

Heat oven to 350°F. Spray a 10-inch quiche pan or pie pan with cooking spray.

With a food processor, use slicing disk to thinly slice apple wedges. Layer apple slices (about 3 1/2 cups) into prepared pan.

Put oil, egg substitute, milk, yogurt, sugar, spices, lemon juice and extracts into food processor. Process until smooth, scraping sides once or twice. Add flours and pulse 3 or 4 times until flours are incorporated, occasionally scraping sides. Do not overmix. Pour mixture over apples. Sprinkle with almonds. If mixture does not all fit into prepared pan, spray custard cups with cooking spray and fill with remaining mixture. Bake as directed.

Bake 40 to 45 minutes or until puffed and browned and knife comes out clean when inserted in center. Cool about 15 minutes before serving. Cover and store in refrigerator.   Bring to room temperature before serving.

❖ Try Rome Beauty, Granny Smith, Golden Delicious, Newtown Pippin apples.

EASY & FLAKY
APPLE TURNOVERS

GRANNY SMITH APPLES ARE PERFECT FOR THIS RECIPE
Prep time: 30 min   Bake time: 15 min
Makes: 12   Serving size: 1 Turnover
Exchanges: 1/2 Fruit (1 Carbohydrate Choice)
Analysis per serving: 38 Calories, 9 g Carbohydrate, 1 g Protein,
0 g Fat, 0 mg Cholesterol, 14 mg Sodium, 1 g Fiber

2 1/4	cups peeled, chopped cooking apples (2-3 medium)
1 1/2	tsp lemon juice
3	Tbs sugar
1/2	tsp cinnamon
1/8	tsp nutmeg
1/4	tsp dried lemon peel or grated fresh lemon peel
1	Tbs flour
6	sheets frozen phyllo pastry, thawed

Butter-flavored cooking spray

Preheat oven to 400°F. Spray baking sheet with cooking spray.

In small bowl, combine chopped apples and lemon juice and toss gently.
Stir in sugar, cinnamon, nutmeg and lemon peel; set aside.

Working with one phyllo sheet at a time, cut each sheet lengthwise into 4
(3 1/2-inch wide) strips. Lightly spray each strip with cooking spray. Stack
2 strips, one on top of the other. Spoon 1 Tbs of apple mixture onto left
side of each strip; flatten apple mixture slightly to within 1 inch of end and
fold the left bottom corner over mixture, forming a triangle. Keep folding
back and forth into a triangle to end of strip. Repeat with remaining pastry
and filling.

Place triangles, seam side down, on prepared baking sheet. Lightly spray
tops with cooking spray. Bake for 15 minutes or until golden brown. Serve
warm.

IMPOSSIBLE
BERRY PIE

A CRUSTLESS BERRY PIE

Prep time: 5 min	Bake time: 45 min
Serves: 10	Serving size: 1 Slice, 1/10 Portion

Exchanges: 1 Starch, 1 Lean meat, 1 Fat (1 Carbohydrate Choice)
Analysis per serving: 180 Calories, 20 g Carbohydrate, 9 g Protein,
7 g Fat, 2 mg Cholesterol, 115 mg Sodium, 1 g Fiber

2	**cups fresh berries, washed & drained (strawberries, raspberries or blueberries)**
1	**13-ounce can evaporated skim milk**
1/4	**cup sugar**
1	**tsp butter extract**
1/4	**cup whole-wheat flour**
1/4	**cup all-purpose flour**
1	**tsp vanilla extract**
1	**cup egg substitute**
1/4	**cup olive or canola oil**
1/4	**tsp almond extract**
1/3	**cup coconut (optional)**

Preheat oven to 350°F. Spray a 10-inch pie plate with cooking spray. Place berries of your choice in pie plate; set aside.

Shake evaporated milk and pour into food processor or blender. Add sugar, butter extract, flours, vanilla, egg substitute, oil and almond extract; process until smooth, scraping sides. Add coconut, if using, and pulse 2 times.

Pour mixture over fruit and bake 45 to 50 minutes or until golden brown and knife inserted in center comes out clean. Cool on rack about 30 minutes and refrigerate about 1 hour before serving. Cover and refrigerate leftovers.

❖ Can use 2 cups frozen berries; do not thaw.

BLUEBERRY COBBLER

QUICK TO FIX — BAKE WHILE PREPARING DINNER
Prep time: 10 min   Bake time: 40 min
Serves: 6   Serving size: 1/6 Portion
Exchanges: 1/2 Starch, 1 Fruit and 1 Fat (2 Carbohydrate Choices)
Analysis per serving: 156 Calories, 26 g Carbohydrate, 3 g Protein,
5 g Fat, 0 mg Cholesterol, 118 mg Sodium, 2 g Fiber

2	**cups (1 pint) blueberries, washed & drained**
1/3	**cup all-purpose flour**
1/3	**cup whole-wheat flour**
1/4	**cup sugar**
1	**tsp dried lemon peel or freshly grated lemon peel**
1 1/2	**tsp baking powder**
2/3	**cup skim milk**
2	**Tbs olive or canola oil**

Preheat oven to 350°F. Spray a 1-quart casserole with cooking spray. Put blueberries in prepared casserole.

In a bowl, use a wooden spoon or a rubber spatula to mix flours, sugar, lemon peel and baking powder. Add milk and oil; mix well.

Spoon mixture over blueberries and bake 40 to 45 minutes or until top is browned. Serve warm.

❖ 2 cups frozen blueberries (do not thaw) can be substituted for fresh blueberries.

BLUEBERRY MERINGUE PIE

MAKE ON A DRY DAY OR THE MERINGUE WILL ABSORB WATER AND FLOP
Prep time: 10 min   Bake time: 35 min
Serves: 8   Serving size: 1 Slice, 1/8 Portion
Exchanges: 1 Starch, 1 Fruit and 1 1/2 Fat (2 Carbohydrate Choices)
Analysis per serving: 202 Calories, 29 g Carbohydrate, 4 g Protein,
7 g Fat, 0 mg Cholesterol, 135 mg Sodium, 3 g Fiber (with crust)

2	large egg whites at room temperature
1/8	tsp cream of tartar
2	Tbs sugar
3	cups fresh blueberries, washed & well drained or frozen & well drained
1	tsp dried lemon peel or fresh grated lemon peel
1	EASY PIE CRUST (page 182), baked

Preheat oven to 400°F.

In large bowl, using electric mixer at high speed, beat egg whites until frothy; beat in cream of tartar and beat until soft peaks form. Gradually beat in sugar at high speed and beat until stiff peaks form, scraping sides of bowl occasionally. Using a rubber spatula, gently fold in blueberries and lemon peel. Spoon into baked pie shell. Sprinkle with topping.

Topping

1/4	cup whole-wheat flour
1/4	cup old-fashioned oats
2	Tbs sugar
1/4	tsp cinnamon
1/4	tsp nutmeg
3	Tbs light margarine or light butter, chilled & thinly sliced

In small bowl, combine flour, oatmeal, sugar and spices. With pastry blender or two knives scissor-fashion, cut in margarine until consistency of fine crumbs. Sprinkle over blueberry mixture.

Bake for 20 minutes. Cover loosely with aluminum foil and continue baking for 15 minutes. Cool on rack about 1 hour before serving. Cover leftovers and refrigerate.

BLUEBERRY NECTARINE PIE

THE CRUST IS ON THE TOP — THE FILLING ON THE BOTTOM
Prep time: 15 min   Bake time: 40 min
Serves: 8   Serving size: 1 Slice, 1/8 Portion
Exchanges: 1/2 Starch, 1 Fruit and 1 Fat (2 Carbohydrate Choices)
Analysis per serving: 152 Calories, 25 g Carbohydrate, 4 g Protein,
4 g Fat, 12 mg Cholesterol, 75 mg Sodium, 2 g Fiber

2	cups (1 pint) fresh blueberries, washed & drained
1	large ripe nectarine, washed & chopped
3	Tbs instant tapioca
3	Tbs sugar, divided
1	EASY PIE CRUST, (page 182), unbaked and refrigerated

Skim milk to glaze

Preheat oven to 400°F. Spray a 9-inch pie plate.

In a medium bowl, mix blueberries, chopped nectarine, tapioca and 2 Tbs sugar. Stir to combine and spoon into prepared pie plate.

Use a rolling pin to roll out pastry between 2 pieces of waxed paper or plastic wrap to a circle 1-inch bigger than pie pan. Remove 1 sheet of waxed paper and place pastry, paper side up on top of filling. Center dough and peel off waxed paper. Using the prongs of a fork, crimp the edge to seal. Trim the edges and brush the pie crust with milk and sprinkle with remaining 1 Tbs of sugar.

Bake 40 to 50 minutes. If crust browns too quickly, cover loosely with aluminum foil. Cool on rack about 1 hour before serving. Cover and refrigerate leftovers.

❖ 2 cups frozen blueberries (do not thaw) can be substituted for fresh blueberries.

STRAWBERRY RHUBARB PIE

STRAWBERRIES AND RHUBARB — A PERFECT COMBINATION
Prep time: 10 min   Bake time: 1 hr
Serves: 8   Serving size: 1 Slice, 1/8 Portion
Exchanges: 1 Starch, 1/2 Fruit and 2 1/2 Fat (2 Carbohydrate Choices)
Analysis per serving: 272 Calories, 26 g Carbohydrate, 4 g Protein,
11 g Fat, 0 mg Cholesterol, 76 mg Sodium, 4 g Fat

1	**EASY PIE CRUST (page 182), unbaked**
1/2	**tsp butter extract**
1	**pound rhubarb stems, washed & cut into 1-inch chunks**
1/2	**tsp almond extract**
1/4	**tsp cinnamon**
2	**cups (1 pint) fresh strawberries, washed, hulled & sliced**
1/8	**tsp nutmeg**
3	**Tbs sugar**

Preheat oven to 400°F.

In medium bowl, mix all ingredients and spoon into unbaked pie shell.
Sprinkle with topping:

Topping

1/4	**cup whole-wheat flour**
1/4	**tsp nutmeg**
1	**Tbs brown sugar**
1/4	**cup old-fashioned oatmeal**
1/4	**tsp butter extract**
1/4	**cup chopped nuts (optional)**
1/4	**cup olive or canola oil**
1/4	**tsp cinnamon**

In the same bowl, mix all ingredients and sprinkle over filled pie crust.

Bake 10 minutes at 400°F. Reduce oven temperature to 350°F and bake
30 minutes or until browned. If crust browns too quickly, cover edges with
aluminum foil. Cool on rack about 30 minutes. Cover and refrigerate
leftovers.

To prevent a soggy crust, brush unbaked pie crust with a beaten egg
white; let dry for 5 minutes. Proceed as directed.

PEACH HARVEST PIE

ALMOND EXTRACT IS THE SPECIAL INGREDIENT IN THIS DELICIOUS PIE
Prep time: 15 min   Bake time: 45 min
Serves: 8   Serving size: 1 Slice, 1/8 Portion
Exchanges: 1 Starch, 1 Fruit and 2 Fat (2 Carbohydrate Choices)
Fat Analysis per serving: 229 Calories, 32 g Carbohydrate, 4 g Protein,
9 g Fat, 0 mg Cholesterol, 74 mg Sodium, 4 g Fiber

1	Tbs sugar
1/2	tsp cinnamon
1/4	tsp nutmeg
2	Tbs instant tapioca
6	cups peeled & thinly sliced peaches (about 8)
	or 3 16-ounce cans juice-packed sliced peaches, drained,
1	Tbs lemon juice
1/4	tsp almond extract
1	EASY PIE CRUST (page 182), unbaked
1	egg white, beaten (optional)

Preheat oven to 425°F.

In large bowl, combine sugar, cinnamon and tapioca; add sliced peaches and mix well. Add lemon juice and almond extract; mix well. To prevent a soggy crust, it is suggested to brush unbaked pie crust with a beaten egg white; and allow to dry for 5 minutes. Spoon filling into crust.   Sprinkle with topping.

Topping

1/4	cup whole-wheat flour
1/2	tsp cinnamon
1/4	cup old-fashioned oats
1	Tbs brown sugar
1	Tbs sugar
3	Tbs olive or canola oil
1/4	cup chopped nuts (optional)

In small bowl, combine all ingredients until crumbly; sprinkle over filled pie crust.   Bake for 15 minutes at 425°F. Reduce oven temperature to 350°F and bake 30 to 35 minutes or until browned and peach filling is soft. If top browns too quickly, cover with aluminum foil. Cool about 1 hour before serving. Cover and refrigerate leftovers.

❖ To peel peaches, plunge peaches into boiling water for 30 seconds, drain and run under cold water; drain. Peel should slide off.

SUMMER FRUIT PIE

A NO-BAKE FRUIT PIZZA
Prep time: 15 min   Chill time: 4 hrs
Serves: 8   Serving size: 1 Slice, 1/8 Portion
Exchanges: 1/2 Starch, 1 Fruit and 1 Fat (2 Carbohydrate Choices)
Analysis per serving: 165 Calories, 27 g Carbohydrate, 4 g Protein,
4 g Fat, 0 mg Cholesterol, 86 mg Sodium, 2 g Fiber

1	8-ounce can juice-packed pineapple chunks
1	envelope unflavored gelatin
1/4	cup cold water
1/4	cup sugar
3/4	cup plain nonfat yogurt
1	tsp vanilla extract
1	EASY PIE CRUST (page 182), baked
1/2	tsp cinnamon
1	large fresh peach, peeled & thinly sliced
3/4	cup fresh sliced strawberries
3/4	cup fresh blueberries, washed & drained

Drain pineapple juice into a small bowl or a 2-cup measuring cup; reserve pineapple chunks. Add enough water to measure 1 cup.

In 1-cup glass measuring cup, sprinkle gelatin over 1/4 cup of cold water; let sit 1 minute to soften. Microwave 1 minute; stir to dissolve gelatin. Pour gelatin into pineapple juice and stir in sugar. Refrigerate about 1 hour or until syrupy.

Reserve 1/4 cup of pineapple-gelatin mixture for glaze. Mix remainder with yogurt and vanilla. Spread yogurt mixture over bottom of baked pie shell. Sprinkle with cinnamon.

Attractively arrange drained pineapple chunks, sliced peach, strawberries and blueberries over yogurt mixture. Gently brush fruit with reserved pineapple-gelatin mixture. Refrigerate, covered, at least 4 hours or overnight before serving.

CREAMY PEACH PIE

TASTY AND SO SIMPLE TO PREPARE!
Prep time: 5 min   Chill time: 3 hrs
Serves: 8   Serving size: 1 Slice, 1/8 Portion
Exchanges: 1 Starch (1 Carbohydrate Choice)
Analysis per serving: 78 Calories, 14 g Carbohydrate, 5 g Protein,
0 g Fat, 5 mg Cholesterol, 162 mg Sodium, 1 g Fiber

2	Tbs graham cracker crumbs
1	envelope gelatin
1/4	cup cold water
1	16-ounce can juice-packed peaches, drained
1	8-ounce package nonfat cream cheese, cubed
2	Tbs sugar
1/2	tsp almond extract

Spray an 8-inch pie pan with cooking spray, and sprinkle bottom and sides with graham cracker crumbs. Set aside.

In food processor without blade or in blender, add water and sprinkle gelatin over water. Let stand 2 minutes. Meanwhile, drain peaches over a glass measuring cup or a small microwaveable bowl. Microwave peach juice on High for 2 1/2 minutes or until very hot. Put blade into food processor. With machine running, pour hot juice into food processor and process until gelatin is completely dissolved, about 1 or 2 minutes. Scrape sides.

Add drained peaches, cream cheese cubes, sugar and almond extract. Process until blended, about 1 minute, scraping sides occasionally.

Pour into prepared pan and chill 3 hours or until firm. If desired, garnish with additional peach slices and a light sprinkling of graham cracker crumbs.

OLD-FASHIONED PEACH COBBLER

CAN USE 2 16-OUNCE CANS JUICE-PACKED PEACHES, SLICED
Prep time: 15 min   Bake time: 40 min
Serves: 8   Serving size: 1/8 Portion
Exchanges: 1 Starch, 1 Fruit and 1/2 Fat (2 Carbohydrate Choices)
Analysis per serving: 152 Calories, 28 g Carbohydrate, 4 g Protein,
3 g Fat, 7 mg Cholesterol, 201 mg Sodium, 3 g Fiber

2	Tbs brown sugar
1/2	tsp cinnamon
1	tsp dried lemon peel or grated fresh lemon peel
1	Tbs lemon juice
4	cups peeled, sliced peaches (5 or 6 medium)
1/2	cup whole-wheat flour
3/4	cup all-purpose flour
1	Tbs baking powder
4	Tbs light margarine or light butter, softened
2	Tbs sugar
2	large egg whites
1/2	cup skim milk
1/2	tsp vanilla extract

Preheat oven to 375°F. Spray an 8-inch square pan with cooking spray.

In medium bowl, combine brown sugar, cinnamon, lemon peel and juice. Add peaches, toss to mix. Transfer to prepared pan. Bake 10 minutes. Meanwhile, combine flours and baking powder in a small bowl; set aside.

In medium bowl, with electric mixer at medium speed, beat margarine and sugar until light and fluffy. Beat in egg whites at medium speed until blended; scrape bowl.

Using a rubber spatula, add dry ingredients alternately with milk and vanilla, beginning and ending with dry ingredients until blended; do not overmix.

Remove peaches from oven and drop spoonfuls of batter over peach mixture; spread gently. Bake 25 to 30 minutes more or until top is golden brown. Serve warm.

❖ To peel peaches plunge peaches into boiling for 30 seconds, drain and run under cold water; drain. Peel should slide off.

PEACH RASPBERRY COBBLER

CAN ALSO BE PREPARED WITH FROZEN PEACHES AND RASPBERRIES
Prep time: 20 min   Bake time: 20 min
Serves: 8   Serving size: 1 Slice, 1/8 Portion
Exchanges: 1 Starch, 1 Fruit and 1/2 Fat (2 Carbohydrate Choices)
Analysis per serving: 159 Calories, 30 g Carbohydrate, 4 g Protein,
3 g Fat, 32 mg Cholesterol, 82 mg Sodium, 5 g Fiber

2	Tbs sugar
1	Tbs cornstarch
2	Tbs water
4	cups peeled, sliced fresh peaches (6 medium)
1	tsp dried lemon peel or grated fresh lemon peel
1	tsp lemon juice
2	cups fresh raspberries, washed & drained

Topping

1/2	cup all-purpose flour
1/2	cup whole-wheat flour
2	Tbs sugar
1	tsp baking powder
1/2	tsp cinnamon
3	Tbs light butter or light margarine
1	large egg, beaten or 1/4 cup egg substitute, shaken
3	Tbs skim milk

Preheat oven to 400°F. Spray a shallow 2-quart casserole with cooking spray.

In a large microwavable bowl, combine sugar and cornstarch. Add water and mix well. Stir in peach slices, lemon peel and lemon juice. Microwave on High for 9 minutes or until thickened and bubbly, stirring every 3 minutes. Gently fold in raspberries. Microwave 1 1/2 minutes, stir gently and microwave another minute. Spoon into prepared casserole.

While fruit is cooking, prepare topping. In small bowl, stir together flours, 2 Tbs sugar, baking powder and cinnamon. Cut in butter or margarine with pastry blender or two knives scissor-fashion until mixture resembles coarse crumbs. Mix beaten egg and milk together and add to flour mixture, stirring just to moisten.

Immediately drop dough into 6 mounds onto hot fruit mixture. Bake 20 to 25 minutes or until a toothpick inserted into topping comes out clean. Serve warm with WHIPPED TOPPING (page 79).

ITALIAN PLUM TART

ITALIAN PLUMS RESEMBLE PLUMP PRUNES
Prep time: 10 min   Bake time: 40 min
Serves: 8   Serving size: 1 Slice, 1/8 Portion
Exchanges: 1 Starch, 1 Fruit and 1/2 Fat (2 Carbohydrate Choices)
Analysis per serving: 161 Calories, 28 g Carbohydrate, 6 g Protein,
3 g Fat, 8 mg Cholesterol, 80 mg Sodium, 2 g Fiber

3	cups (1 pound) Italian plums, washed, halved & pitted (12-14 plums)
2/3	cup evaporated skim milk (shake before measuring)
2	Tbs sugar
1/2	cup egg substitute
1	tsp almond extract
1	9-inch TART SHELL (page 185), baked

Preheat oven to 350°F. Spray cooking spray on baking sheet large enough to hold baked tart shell. Cover outside of tart pan with 2 layers of aluminum foil to prevent leakage.

Thinly slice each plum half . You should have about 3 cups. Arrange fruit in tart shell, slightly overlapping, to cover bottom; place tart on prepared baking sheet.

In 4-cup glass measuring cup, use a whisk to beat evaporated milk, sugar, egg substitute and extract until blended. Place baking sheet with tart in oven and carefully pour mixture over plums.

Bake 40 to 45 minutes or until custard is set and knife inserted in center comes out clean. Cool about 1 hour before serving. Remove pan rim to serve. Cover and refrigerate leftovers.

❖ If Italian plums are not available, use 3 cups fruit of your choice.

CRUSTLESS PUMPKIN PIE

MAPLE EXTRACT IS THE SPECIAL INGREDIENT
Prep time: 5 min   Bake time: 35 min
Serves: 10   Serving size: 1 Slice, 1/10 Portion
Exchanges: 1 Skim Milk (1 Carbohydrate Choice)
Analysis per serving: 93 Calories, 16 g Carbohydrate, 6 g Protein,
1 g Fat, 2 mg Cholesterol, 131 mg Sodium, 2 g Fiber

1/2	cup egg substitute
1	13-ounce can evaporated skim milk
1	16-ounce can pumpkin (NOT pie filling)
	or 2 cups fresh pureed pumpkin
1/2	cup reduced-fat buttermilk baking mix
	(preferably whole-wheat)
1	tsp cinnamon
1/2	tsp nutmeg
1/2	tsp ginger
1/4	tsp cloves
1/4	tsp allspice
1/2	tsp maple extract
3	Tbs brown sugar

Preheat oven to 400°F. Spray a 10-inch pie plate with cooking spray.

In food processor, process egg substitute. Shake evaporated milk and add to processor along with remaining ingredients. Process until smooth, scraping sides occasionally. Pour into prepared pie plate. Use sprayed custard cups to hold any extra filling, and bake with pie.

Bake 35 to 40 minutes or until set. A pick inserted in center should come out clean. Do not over bake. Cool on rack about 30 minutes and refrigerate about 2 hours or overnight before serving. Serve with WHIPPED TOPPING (page 79) or EASY FAT-FREE TOPPING (page 80).

DATE CHIFFON PIE FILLING

A LIGHT AND NATURALLY SWEET PIE
Prep time: 10 min   Chill time: 2 hrs
Serves: 8   Serving size: 1 Slice, 1/8 Portion
Exchanges: 1/2 Starch, 1/2 Lean meat and 1 Fruit (2 Carbohydrate Choices)
Analysis per serving: 130 Calories, 27 g Carbohydrate, 4 g Protein,
1 g Fat, 54 mg Cholesterol, 71 mg Sodium, 2 g Fiber (without crust)

4	**Tbs sugar, divided**
1	**envelope unflavored gelatin**
1 1/4	**cups orange juice**
2	**large egg yolks, beaten**
1	**cup finely chopped dates**
2	**tsp dried orange peel or grated fresh lemon peel**
1	**cup plain nonfat yogurt**
2	**large egg whites**
1/8	**tsp salt**
1/2	**tsp cinnamon**
1/4	**tsp allspice**
1	**9-inch baked pie shell of your choice**

In 4-cup glass measuring cup, use a whisk to combine 2 Tbs sugar, gelatin, orange juice and egg yolks. Microwave on Medium/High for 6 minutes, stirring every 2 minutes, until slightly thickened. Use a rubber spatula to stir in dates, orange peel and yogurt; mix well. Refrigerate about 1 hour or until mixture begins to set.

In medium bowl, with electric mixer at high speed, beat egg whites, which have been at room temperature, with salt and remaining 2 Tbs sugar and spices until stiff peaks form when beaters are lifted. Do not over beat. Use a rubber spatula to gently fold stiff egg whites into gelatin mixture until no white streaks remain and batter is well blended.

Spoon into baked pie shell. Chill at least 2 hours or until firm.

LEMON CHIFFON PIE

A WONDERFUL SUMMER PIE — SO COOL & REFRESHING
Prep time: 15 min   Chill time: 6 hr
Serves: 8   Serving size: 1 Slice, 1/8 Portion
Exchanges: 1 Starch, 1/2 Lean meat and 1 Fat (1 Carbohydrate Choice)
Analysis per serving: 151 Calories, 15 g Carbohydrate, 6 g Protein,
8 g Fat, 80 mg Cholesterol, 120 mg Sodium, 0 g Fiber

Crust

1	cup graham cracker crumbs
3	Tbs olive or canola oil

In small bowl, mix ingredients and press firmly onto bottom and part way up sides of 9-inch pie plate; chill about 1 hour.

Filling

1	envelope unflavored gelatin
4	Tbs sugar, divided
1 1/2	cups skim milk, divided
3	large eggs yolks
1/4	cup lemon juice
2	tsp dried lemon peel or 1 tsp grated fresh lemon peel

Pasteurized dried egg white for 3 egg whites
Water   (see page 13)

In a 4-cup glass measuring cup, mix gelatin, 2 Tbs sugar and 1/2 cup milk; let stand 1 minute.

In a medium bowl, use a whisk to beat remaining 1 cup milk with egg yolks; stir into gelatin mixture. Microwave Medium/High for 5 or 6 minutes, stirring every 2 minutes, until gelatin is completely dissolved. Stir in juice and peel. Chill, about 1 hour, stirring occasionally, until mixture mounds when dropped from spoon.

In medium bowl, with electric mixer at high speed, beat dried egg whites and water until soft peaks form. Gradually beat in remaining 2 Tbs sugar until stiff peaks form when batter is lifted with a rubber spatula. Use rubber spatula to gently fold beaten whites into lemon mixture until no white streaks remain and mixture is well mixed.

Spoon into prepared crust. Chill until firm, 6 hours or overnight.

CHOCOLATE MERINGUE PIE

IT'S SO GOOD, YOU WON'T BELIEVE IT'S LOW-FAT
Prep time: 20 min   Cook time: 35 min   Chill time: 3 hrs
Serves: 8   Serving size: 1 Slice, 1/8 Portion
Exchanges: 1 Skim milk, 1 Starch and 1 Fat (2 Carbohydrate Choices)
Analysis per serving: 202 Calories, 32 g Carbohydrate, 8 g Protein,
6 g Fat, 27 mg Cholesterol, 141 mg Sodium, 2 g Fiber

1/3	cup cocoa
1/4	cup sugar
1/4	cup cornstarch, divided
2	cups skim milk
1	large egg or 1/4 cup egg substitute
2	tsp vanilla extract
Pasteurized dried egg white for 3 egg whites	
Water	(see page 13)
1/4	tsp cream of tartar
2	Tbs sugar
1	9-inch TASTY FLAKEY PIE CRUST (page 183), baked

In 4-cup glass measuring cup, combine cocoa, 1/4 cup sugar, and 3 Tbs of cornstarch; gradually add milk, stirring with wire whisk until well blended.

Microwave 6 to 8 minutes at Medium/High, stirring every 2 minutes, or until mixture boils. Put egg in 1-cup glass measuring cup; use a small whisk or a fork to beat egg slightly. Remove cocoa mixture from microwave and gradually stir 1/4 cup of hot cocoa mixture into beaten egg; add egg mixture to cocoa mixture; stir to blend. Microwave High for 1 minute or until thickened and bubbly. Stir in vanilla. Cover with plastic wrap and set aside.

Preheat oven 325°F. In medium bowl, with electric mixer at high speed, beat dried egg whites, water, remaining tablespoon of cornstarch and cream of tartar until foamy. Gradually beat in 2 Tbs sugar at high speed, one tablespoon at a time, until stiff peaks form when batter is lifted with rubber spatula. Do not over beat.

Remove plastic wrap from chocolate filling and stir; pour into cooled pie shell. Gently spread meringue evenly over filling, sealing to edge of pastry. Bake 25 minutes or until lightly browned. Cool on rack for 30 minutes and refrigerate 3 hours or until set before serving.

FUDGEY CHEESE PIE

THE TASTE OF A FUDGESCICLE IN A PIE — BEST IF MADE THE NIGHT BEFORE
Prep time: 5 min   Cook time: 2 hrs   Chill time: 4 hrs
Serves: 8   Serving size: 1 Slice, 1/8 Portion
Exchanges: 1/2 Lean meat, 1 Starch and 1 Fat (1 Carbohydrate Choice)
Analysis per serving: 158 Calories, 20 g Carbohydrate, 6 g Protein,
7 g Fat, 1 mg Cholesterol, 248 mg Sodium, 1 g Fiber

Crust

1	**cup graham cracker crumbs**
3	**Tbs olive or canola oil**
1	**Tbs cocoa**

Spray 9-inch pie pan with cooking spray. In a medium bowl, combine all ingredients. Pat into bottom and part way up sides of prepared pie pan; set aside.

Filling

1	**cup nonfat ricotta or cottage cheese**
3/4	**cup skim milk**
2	**tsp cornstarch**
1/8	**tsp salt**
3	**tsp vanilla extract, divided**
5	**Tbs sugar, divided**
1/2	**cup egg substitute**
1	**tsp instant coffee powder**
4	**Tbs cocoa**

Preheat oven to 350°F.

In food processor or blender, combine ricotta, milk, cornstarch, salt, 1 tsp of vanilla and 2 Tbs sugar. Process until smooth, scraping sides. Add egg substitute, process until smooth, scraping sides. Pour 1 cup of mixture into prepared crust.

Bake 20 minutes or until firm. Add remaining 3 Tbs sugar, 2 tsp vanilla, instant coffee and cocoa to the ricotta mixture; process to combine until blended. Scrape sides and pour chocolate mixture over baked vanilla layer.

Bake an additional 20 minutes or until set. Turn off oven and leave door slightly ajar for 1 hour. Remove to rack for about 1 hour. Cover and chill at least 4 hours or overnight before serving. If desired, top with WHIPPED TOPPING (page 79) or EASY FAT-FREE TOPPING (page 80).

STRAWBERRY YOGURT PIE FILLING

FROZEN STRAWBERRIES WILL SPEED UP THE THICKENING PROCESS
Prep time: 10 min   Chill time: 1-3 hrs
Serves: 8   Serving size: 1 Slice, 1/8 Portion
Exchanges: 1 Fruit (1 Carbohydrate Choice)
Analysis per serving: 51 Calories, 11 g Carbohydrate, 2 g Protein,
0 g Fat, 0 mg Cholesterol, 13 mg Sodium, 1 g Fiber (without crust)

2	Tbs unsweetened apple juice concentrate, thawed
2	Tbs cold water
1	envelope unflavored gelatin
1/3	cup boiling water
1	Tbs sugar
1	medium ripe banana, sliced into 1-inch pieces
3/4	cup plain nonfat yogurt
1	tsp vanilla extract
2	cups whole natural frozen strawberries (do not thaw) or 2 cups fresh berries washed, drained & halved
1	MERINGUE CRUST (page 180) or FAT-FREE PIE CRUST (page 186) baked

In a 1-cup glass measuring cup, combine juice concentrate and cold water. Sprinkle with gelatin and let sit for 5 minutes until gelatin is softened; stir. Add boiling water; stir to dissolve gelatin.

In food processor or blender, combine gelatin mixture, sugar, banana chunks, yogurt and vanilla; process until smooth, scraping sides occasionally, for about 1 minute. Add strawberries, a few at a time, and process until strawberries are pureed and mixture is smooth, about 1 minute. Scrape sides occasionally.

Pour into a medium bowl; cover and refrigerate at least 1-3 hours or until thickened and firm. About an hour before serving, stir thickened strawberry mixture and pour into baked, cooled pie crust. Refrigerate about an hour before serving. Best served the same day as it's made.

BANANA CREAM TART

STRAWBERRIES, PEACHES OR OTHER FRUIT CAN BE SUBSTITUTED
Prep time: 10 min   Cook time: 1 hr
Serves: 8   Serving size: 1 Slice, 1/8 Portion
Exchanges: 1 Starch, 1 Fruit and 1/2 Fat (2 Carbohydrate Choices)
Analysis per serving: 161 Calories, 30 g Carbohydrate, 4 g Protein,
3 g Fat, 9 mg Cholesterol, 61 mg Sodium, 2 g Fiber (with tart shell)

1	recipe SIMPLE VANILLA PUDDING (page 200)
2	medium ripe bananas
1	9-inch TART SHELL (page 185), baked
	or 9-inch pie shell, baked

Prepare SIMPLE VANILLA PUDDING according to recipe directions.
Cool.

Thinly slice bananas and stir into pudding. Spoon into cooled pie shell.
Chill at least 1 hour or until firm. Remove sides of tart pan; leave tart on
pan bottom and place on plate to serve.

BAKED MERINGUE CRUST (page 180) or FAT-FREE PIE CRUST (page
186) are also perfect for this pie.

DELIGHTFUL PUMPKIN APPLE PIE

TWO FANTASTIC PIES IN ONE
Prep time: 15 min   Bake time: 45 min
Serves: 8   Serving size: 1 Slice, 1/8 Portion
Exchanges: 1 Starch, 1/2 Fruit and 1 Fat (2 Carbohydrate Choices)
Analysis per serving: 163 Calories, 27 g Carbohydrate, 5 g Protein,
5 g Fat, 27 mg Cholesterol, 38 mg Sodium, 4 g Fiber

1	OATMEAL CRUST (page 181) or EASY PIE CRUST (page 182), unbaked
1	egg white, beaten
2	cups cooking apples, peeled and thinly sliced (2 medium)
2	Tbs brown sugar
2	Tbs all-purpose flour
1/2	tsp cinnamon
1/2	tsp ginger
1/8	tsp cloves
2	cups (16-ounce can) pumpkin (NOT pie filling)
2/3	cup evaporated skim milk, shaken
1	large egg or 1/4 cup egg substitute

Preheat oven 425°F. Brush beaten egg white over crust. Reserve remaining egg white. Let crust dry while preparing filling. The egg brush will prevent a soggy crust.

In a large bowl, combine sliced apples, brown sugar, flour and cinnamon until well blended. Spoon into prepared pie crust; set aside.

In same bowl, use a whisk to combine ginger, cloves, pumpkin, skimmed evaporated milk, egg and reserved egg white (which was used to brush crust) until well blended. Pour pumpkin mixture over apples in pie crust. Bake at 425°F for 15 minutes. Reduce oven temperature to 350°F and bake 30 to 35 minutes or until a knife inserted in center comes out clean. Cool about 30 minutes before serving. Store, covered, in refrigerator.

❖ Try Granny Smith, Rome Beauty or Golden Delicious apples.

BAKLAVA

CARBOHYDRATE & FAT CONTENT IS LOWER THAN IN TRADITIONAL BAKLAVA
Prep time: 15 min   Bake time: 30 min
Makes: 24   Serving size: 1
Exchanges: 1/2 Starch
Analysis per serving: 38 Calories, 4 g Carbohydrate, 0 g Protein,
2 g Fat, 2 mg Cholesterol, 15 mg Sodium, 0 g Fiber

1	cup water
1	medium apple, peeled, cored & chopped
1/2	cup raisins
1	tsp cinnamon
3	Tbs light butter or light margarine, melted
3	Tbs olive or canola oil
6	sheets phyllo dough

In 4-cup glass measuring cup, combine water, apple, raisins and cinnamon. Microwave on High for 5 minutes; stir and cook Medium/High for 5 minutes. Stir; let rest 1 minute. Transfer fruit to small bowl with slotted spoon. Microwave liquid on Medium/High for 3 minutes; stir, microwave Medium/High for 2 or 3 minutes or until reduced to a thin syrup.

Preheat oven to 375°F. Spray a 13x9x2-inch pan with cooking spray. Combine melted butter and oil. Place 1 sheet of phyllo in prepared pan; brush lightly with butter/oil mixture. Repeat with second sheet and brush. Lay third sheet but do not brush. Spoon fruit over phyllo and spread evenly over phyllo. Repeat layering remaining phyllo and brushing lightly with butter/oil mixture.

Use a knife to push edges of phyllo down along sides of pan; score top into diamonds. Brush again with butter/oil mixture. If desired, spray butter flavored cooking spray over baklava.

Bake 30 minutes or until lightly brown. Cool on rack for about 30 minutes and pour reserved syrup over baklava. Let baklava absorb syrup before cutting into diamond shapes. Store in covered container or freeze up to 3 months. Defrost before serving.

MERINGUE CRUST

SIMILAR TO A PAVLOVA
Prep time: 10 min   Bake time: 3 hrs
Makes: 9-inch pie shell   Serving size: 1/8 portion, 8 Servings
Exchanges: 1/2 Fruit (1 Carbohydrate Choice)
Analysis per serving: 30 Calories, 6 g Carbohydrate, 1 g Protein,
0 g Fat, 0 mg Cholesterol, 94 mg Sodium, 0 g Fiber

3	large egg whites at room temperature
1/4	tsp salt
1/4	tsp cream tartar
1/2	tsp almond extract
1/4	cup sugar

Preheat oven to 300°F. Have a 9-inch pie plate ready.

In large bowl, using electric mixer at high speed, beat egg whites, salt, cream of tartar and extract until soft peaks form. Gradually add sugar, one tablespoon at a time, beating until stiff peaks form when beaters are lifted.

Spread mixture into an ungreased 9-inch pie plate, forming a hollow in the center and building meringue up sides. Bake for 1 hour. Turn oven off, leave oven door closed, and cool pie shell in oven 2 hours or until dry.

Spoon filling of your choice into pie shell just before serving.

❖ Do not make on a wet or humid day since the meringue tends to draw moisture from the air. The results will be a soggy crust.

This pie shell is delicious filled with a mixture of 2 cups berries (such as a combination of strawberries, blueberries, raspberries), 1/2 cup nonfat yogurt cream, 1/2 tsp vanilla extract, 1/4 tsp almond extract and 2 Tbs sugar.

MERINGUE CRUST can be prepared up to 2 days ahead and stored loosely covered at room temperature. Fill just before serving.

OATMEAL CRUST

A TASTY PIE CRUST WITH APPLE OR PUMPKIN FILLING
Prep time: 5 min   Bake time: 8 min
Makes: 9-inch crust   Serving size: 1/8 Portion, 8 servings
Exchanges: 1/2 Starch and 1/2 Fat (1 Carbohydrate Choice)
Analysis per serving: 82 Calories, 11 g Carbohydrate, 2 g Protein,
4 g Fat, 0 mg Cholesterol, 2 mg Sodium, 1 g Fiber

1/2	cup old-fashioned oats
1/2	cup whole-wheat flour
2	Tbs brown sugar
1/2	tsp cinnamon
2	Tbs olive or canola oil
1	Tbs warm water

Preheat oven 350°F. Have a 9-inch springform pan or a 10-inch pie plate ready.

In medium bowl, combine oatmeal, flour, sugar and cinnamon. Add oil and water and mix well with fork until crumbly.

Pat onto bottom and part way up sides of an ungreased 9-inch springform pan or a 10-inch pie plate. Bake 8 to 10 minutes or until golden brown. Cool on rack before filling.

EASY PIE CRUST

USED IN SEVERAL PIE FILLING RECIPES IN THIS SECTION
Prep time: 10 min   Bake time: 10 min
Makes: 8- or 9-inch crust   Serving size: 1/8 Portion, 8 servings
Exchanges: 1/2 Starch and 1 Fat (1 Carbohydrate Choice)
Analysis per serving: 95 Calories, 11 g Carbohydrate, 2 g Protein,
4 g Fat, 0 mg Cholesterol, 73 mg Sodium, 1 g Fiber

1/2	cup all-purpose flour
1/2	cup whole-wheat flour
1/4	tsp salt
3	Tbs solid vegetable shortening
2	Tbs cold water

In a small bowl, mix flours and salt. Using fork or pastry blender, add
vegetable shortening and mix until crumbly. Using a wooden spoon or
rubber spatula, stir in water until mixture forms a ball. Wrap in plastic
wrap; press to flatten slightly. Refrigerate about 1 hour for easier rolling.

To make in food processor: put flours and salt in food processor. Add
vegetable shortening and pulse until crumbly (3-4 times). Add water and
pulse until a ball forms. Immediately remove, wrap in plastic wrap and
refrigerate about 1 hour for easy rolling.

Place unwrapped dough between 2 pieces of waxed paper or plastic wrap
and use a rolling pin to roll into a 10- or 11-inch circle. Peel off 1 piece of
paper and place paper-side up into 8 or 9-inch pie plate. Press onto
bottom and sides of plate; flute.

To make an unfilled crust: prick bottom and sides with a fork. Bake at
400°F for 10 minutes or until lightly browned. Cool on a rack before filling.

For a filled pie crust: do not prick. Spoon in filling and bake as directed.

❖ If filling crust with a fruit filling, brush unbaked pie crust with a beaten
egg white. If filling unbaked crust, let dry for 5 minutes before filling. If
recipe for a fruit-filled pie calls for a baked crust, brush unbaked crust with
beaten egg white and bake as directed; cool. Proceed with recipe.

TASTY, FLAKEY PIE CRUST

A QUICK FIX PIE CRUST THAT MELTS IN YOUR MOUTH
Prep time: 10 min   Bake time: 14 min
Makes: 9-inch crust   Serving size: 1/8 Portion, 8 Servings
Exchanges: 1/2 Starch and 1 Fat (1 Carbohydrate Choice)
Analysis per serving: 95 Calories, 11 g Carbohydrate, 2 g Protein,
5 g Fat, 0 mg Cholesterol, 73 mg Sodium, 1 g Fiber

1/2	cup whole-wheat flour
1/2	cup all-purpose flour
1/4	tsp salt
3	Tbs solid vegetable shortening
3	Tbs ice water
1	tsp lemon juice

Preheat oven to 425°F. Spray a 9-inch pie plate with cooking spray.

In small bowl, combine flours and salt. Using pastry blender or two knives scissor-fashion, cut in shortening until mixture is crumbly. Combine water and lemon juice. Sprinkle ice water mixture, 1 tablespoon at a time, over surface of flour mixture. Toss with fork until dry ingredients are moistened.

Gently press dough into a 4-inch circle on plastic wrap. Cover with additional plastic wrap and roll dough, still covered, into an 11-inch circle. Place dough in freezer 5 minutes or until plastic wrap can be easily removed.

Remove plastic wrap and fit dough into prepared 9-inch pie plate. Fold edges under and flute; prick bottom and sides of dough with fork. Bake 14 minutes or until lightly browned; cool on rack before filling.

❖ To prevent a soggy crust for a fruit filled pie, brush unbaked pie crust with a beaten egg white. Let dry for about 5 minutes before proceeding with recipe.

ZIP ZAP PIE CRUST

THIS CRUST IS PERFECT FOR FRUIT FILLINGS
Prep time: 45 min   Bake time: 5 min
Makes: 9-inch crust   Serving size: 1/8 Portion, 8 Servings
Exchanges: 1 Fruit and 1 Fat (1 Carbohydrate Choice)
Analysis per serving: 110 Calories, 12 g Carbohydrate, 3 g Protein,
6 g Fat, 0 mg Cholesterol, 80 mg Sodium, 1 g Fiber

1/2	cup whole-wheat flour
1/2	cup all-purpose flour
2	Tbs finely chopped nuts
1/4	tsp salt
3	Tbs solid vegetable shortening
2-3	Tbs apple juice
1	egg white, beaten

Have a 9-inch pie plate ready.

In medium bowl, combine flours, nuts and salt. Using pastry blender or two knives scissor-fashion, cut in shortening until crumbly. Sprinkle with 2 or 3 Tbs apple juice and gently stir with fork until mixture forms ball. Cover with plastic wrap and flatten slightly; refrigerate 30 minutes.

Preheat oven 425°F. Remove plastic wrap. With rolling pin, roll dough between 2 pieces of waxed paper or plastic wrap to 11-inch circle. Remove 1 piece of paper and place in pie plate paper side up. Gently remove paper and press into pie place. Turn edges under and flute. Prick bottom and sides of crust with fork. Brush with a small amount of beaten egg white. Let dry for 5 minutes. Bake 5 minutes or until golden brown. Cool on rack before filling.

TART SHELL

USE FOR BANANA CREAM OR ITALIAN PLUM TARTS
Prep time: 15 min   Bake time: 10 min
Makes: 9-inch shell   Serving size: 1/8 Portion, 8 Servings
Exchanges: 1 Starch and 1/2 Fat (1 Carbohydrate Choice)
Analysis per serving: 90 Calories, 15 g Carbohydrate, 2 g Protein,
3 g Fat, 7 mg Cholesterol, 28 mg Sodium, 1 g Fiber

1/2	cup whole-wheat flour
1/2	cup all-purpose flour
2	Tbs sugar
1/4	cup light margarine or light butter
1-2	Tbs cold water

Have a 9-inch tart pan with removable bottom ready.

In medium bowl, mix flours and sugar. Using pastry blender or two knives scissor-fashion, cut in margarine or butter until crumbly. Sprinkle with 1 Tbs of water and stir with fork until mixture clumps together to form dough. Add remaining 1 Tbs water if necessary. Press dough over bottom and sides of ungreased tart pan. Prick bottom all over with fork. Cover with plastic wrap and chill 1 hour.

Preheat oven to 425°F. Remove tart shell from refrigerator. Put tart pan on baking sheet; bake 10 to 12 minutes or until golden brown. Cool on rack before filling.

FAT-FREE PIE CRUST

NO NEED TO ROLL THIS CRUST — PUDDINGS MAKE GREAT FILLINGS
Prep time: 5 min   Bake time: 15 min
Makes: 1 pie crust   Serving size: 1/8 Portion, 8 Servings
Exchanges: 1/2 Starch
Analysis per serving: 18 Calories, 4 g Carbohydrate, 1 g Protein,
0 g Fat, 0 mg Cholesterol, 21 mg Sodium, 0 g Fiber

6   sheets of phyllo dough (12x17-inches), defrosted
Butter-flavored cooking spray

Preheat oven 350°F.

Spray an 8-, 9- or 10-inch pie plate with butter-flavored cooking spray.
Lay 3 sheets phyllo dough across pie plate with dough hanging over pie
plate on two sides; gently press into pie plate with your fingers. Lay
remaining 3 sheets of phyllo in opposite direction across pie plate,
extending dough; gently press dough with fingers.

Using scissors specifically for food or a very sharp knife, trim dough about
2 inches beyond rim of pie plate. Gently turn dough under leaving a ridge
around rim of pie plate. Pierce bottom and sides of crust with fork.   Spray
pie crust completely and evenly with butter-flavored cooking spray.

If desired, shape phyllo trimmings into decorative shapes, place on baking
sheet and spray with cooking spray. Bake crust and shapes for 15
minutes or until golden brown; cool before filling. Fill cooled pie crust with
pudding and fruit of your choice. Refrigerate at least 1 hour or until set;
garnish with bundles.

❖ This pie crust is best made and served the same day.

Puddings

Kind of fun — creamy and cool — each of these pudding recipes is less than 150 calories per serving with 3 or less grams of fat. Puddings are very versatile. By adding fruit, they make a speedy breakfast. Everyone loves opening their lunch to find a sweet serving of pudding. And who could resist a tempting pudding snack in the afternoon?

Of these, some are tried and true basics, like FABULOUS CHOCOLATE PUDDING and SIMPLE VANILLA PUDDING. FRUITY NOODLE PUDDING is unusual but wonderful. For more elegance, serve ORANGE SOUFFLE or ORANGE HONEY CUSTARD.

We live in the convenience age where puddings can be dumped out of box and whipped instantly. With the pudding recipes in DIABETIC GOODIE BOOK, the investment in longer cooking times is well worth it in the end. They are very low in sugar and fat; they use skim milk, fresh fruits and wholesome rice and tapioca. The ultimate results are that these recipes are tasty, filling and satisfying. Serve them up in tall, parfait glasses — everyone at your table will smile!

FABULOUS CHOCOLATE PUDDING

SO GOOD, YOU'LL NEVER GO BACK TO STORE-BOUGHT PUDDING
Prep time: 10 min   Cook time: 1 hr
Serves: 4   Serving size: 1/2 Cup
Exchanges: 1/2 Skim milk and 1 Starch for pudding and pie (1 Carbohydrate Choice)
Analysis per serving—Pudding/Pie 8 portions: 91/92 Calories, 18/20 g Carbohydrate,
5/4 g Protein, 0/0 g Fat, 2/2 mg Cholesterol, 64/53 mg Sodium, 0/1 g Fiber

2	**cups skim milk, divided**
2	**Tbs cocoa**
2	**Tbs sugar**
2 1/2	**Tbs cornstarch**
2	**tsp vanilla extract**

In a 4-cup glass measuring cup, measure 1 1/2 cups milk. Microwave on High for 3 or 4 minutes or until milk is scalded.

Meanwhile, in a small bowl, combine cocoa, sugar and cornstarch. Use a whisk to stir in remaining 1/2 cup of milk; mix until smooth. Stir cocoa mixture into scalded milk until well blended. Cook on High for 2 minutes, stir and cook another 2 to 3 minutes or until mixture has thickened.

Let rest 1 minute, then stir in vanilla. Spoon into 4 dessert dishes. Chill about 1 hour before serving.

CHOCOLATE PUDDING PIE

1	**baked 8- or 9-inch FAT-FREE PIE CRUST (page 186) or MERINGUE CRUST (page 180)**
2	**medium bananas, thinly sliced**
1	**Tbs orange juice**
1	**recipe FABULOUS CHOCOLATE PUDDING, prepared**

Put sliced bananas in small bowl and add orange juice. Stir to coat so bananas do not turn brown. Arrange bananas over pie crust. Pour pudding over bananas. Chill at least one hour before serving.

❖ For a variation, use SIMPLE VANILLA PUDDING (page 200) for the pie.

STUPENDOUS
STRAWBERRY PUDDING

SO DELICIOUS YOU MAY LIKE THIS PUDDING BETTER THAN FRESH BERRIES
Prep time: 10 min   Cook time: 1 hr
Serves: 8   Serving size: 1/2 Cup
Exchanges: 1 Fruit (1 Carbohydrate Choice)
Analysis per serving: 57 Calories, 11 g Carbohydrate, 3 g Protein,
0 g Fat, 1 mg Cholesterol, 18 mg Sodium, 2 g Fiber

2	envelopes unflavored gelatin
1/2	cup cold water
1	cup skim milk
3	Tbs sugar
1	tsp almond extract
4	cups fresh strawberries, washed & hulled

In a food processor, without a blade, sprinkle gelatin over cold water. Let stand 3 minutes to soften. Meanwhile, heat milk in microwave on High for 3 minutes or heat milk in small pot until almost boiling. Put blade in food processor; add hot milk and process until gelatin is completely dissolved, scraping sides once.

Add sugar and extract. With machine running, gradually drop in strawberries until berries are pureed and incorporated into mixture; scrape sides occasionally . Pour into 8 dessert dishes. Chill about 1 hour or until set.

❖ 4 cups of frozen unsweetened strawberries may be substituted. Pudding will be firm in about 30 minutes. This recipe is a great way to use bruised strawberries. Spray a 4-cup mold with cooking spray and pour in pudding. Cover, refrigerate 2 - 4 hours or until firm. Unmold on serving plate and serve surrounded with additional fresh strawberries.

PUMPKIN PUDDING

ALMOST LIKE PUMPKIN PIE BUT WITHOUT THE CRUST
Prep time: 10 min   Cook time: 5 min
Serves: 6   Serving size: 1/2 Cup
Exchanges: 1 Skim milk (1 Carbohydrate Choice)
Analysis per serving: 87 Calories, 15 g Carbohydrate, 6 g Protein,
0 g Fat, 0 mg Cholesterol, 86 mg Sodium, 1 g Fiber

1/4	**cup cold water**
1	**envelope unflavored gelatin**
1/4	**cup boiling water**
1	**cup cooked or canned pumpkin (NOT pie filling)**
2/3	**cup nonfat dry milk powder**
1/2	**tsp pumpkin pie spice**
1/4	**tsp maple extract**
2	**Tbs sugar**
8	**ice cubes (1 1/2 cups)**

In a food processor without a blade, sprinkle gelatin over cold water. Let rest 3 minutes to soften. Put in blade, add boiling water and process 30 seconds; scrape sides.

Add pumpkin, dry milk powder, pumpkin spice, maple extract and sugar; process until smooth; scrape sides. With machine running, drop in ice cubes, one at a time, and process until cubes are incorporated and mixture is smooth, scraping sides occasionally.

Pour into 6 dessert dishes. Serve immediately or chill until ready to serve.

FRUITY NOODLE PUDDING

REHEAT FOR A TASTY BREAKFAST
Prep time: 10 min   Bake time: 35 min
Serves: 8   Serving size: 1/2 Cup
Exchanges: 1 Starch and 1/2 Fruit (1 Carbohydrate Choice)
Analysis per serving: 104 Calories, 22 g Carbohydrate, 3 g Protein,
1 g Fat, 14 mg Cholesterol, 19 mg Sodium, 1 g Fiber

2	cups wide noodles, cooked and drained
2	apples (about 2 cups), peeled, cored and thinly sliced
1	cup plain nonfat yogurt
2	Tbs lemon juice
1	tsp vanilla extract
2	Tbs brown sugar
1/2	tsp cinnamon
1/4	cup seedless white raisins

Preheat oven to 350°F. Spray a 1 1/2- or 2-quart casserole with cooking spray.

In a large bowl, combine all ingredients, mixing well. Spoon mixture into the prepared casserole; bake 35 to 40 minutes or until top is lightly browned. Serve warm or at room temperature. Store leftovers covered in refrigerator.

TEMPTING
RASPBERRY PUDDING

THIS RECIPE TAKES SOME TIME TO PREPARE BUT IS WORTH THE EFFORT
Prep time: 20 min   Chill time: 3 hrs
Serves: 8   Serving size: 1/2 Cup
Exchanges: 1 Skim milk and 1 Fruit (1 Carbohydrate Choice)
Analysis per serving: 126 Calories, 23 g Carbohydrate, 8 g Protein,
0 g Fat, 0 mg Cholesterol, 166 mg Sodium, 5 g Fiber

2	**envelopes unflavored gelatin**
1/2	**cup cold water**
4	**cups fresh or frozen unsweetened raspberries**
1/4	**cup low-sugar raspberry jam**
1/4	**cup sugar, divided**
1	**cup unsweetened applesauce**
1	**cup nonfat ricotta cheese**

Pasteurized dried egg white for 4 egg whites

Water	**(see page 13)**
1/2	**tsp cream of tartar**

In a small bowl, sprinkle gelatin over cold water. Let stand 3 minutes to soften.

Meanwhile, in a glass 4-cup measuring cup, mix raspberries, jam and 2 Tbs sugar. Microwave on High for 4 minutes, stirring every 2 minutes until mixture comes to a boil. Stir in gelatin mixture until gelatin is completely dissolved; cool 5 minutes.

Press the mixture through a strainer into a large bowl; discard seeds. You should have about 3 cups of mixture. Stir in applesauce. Refrigerate about 1 hour or more, stirring 3 times, or until mixture thickens to consistency of unbeaten egg whites and mounds when dropped from a spoon.

In a food processor, process ricotta cheese until smooth and creamy. Stir into the thickened fruit mixture.

In a medium bowl, beat dried egg white, water and cream of tartar with an electric mixer at high speed until foamy. Gradually add remaining 2 Tbs sugar and continue beating at high speed, scraping sides occasionally until stiff peaks form when lifted with a rubber spatula.

Gently fold stiffly beaten meringue into fruit mixture until no white streaks remain. Spoon into 8 dessert dishes. Chill about 3 hours or until set. If desired, top each dessert with a raspberry.

CREAMY RICE PUDDING

GREAT SERVED FOR BREAKFAST
Prep time: 5 min   Cook time: 40 min
Serves: 10   Serving size: 1/2 Cup
Exchanges: 1 Starch and 1 Fruit (2 Carbohydrate Choices)
Analysis per serving: 138 Calories, 26 g Carbohydrate, 8 g Protein,
1 g Fat, 3 mg Cholesterol, 99 mg Sodium, 1 g Fiber

1	12-ounce can evaporated skim milk
2 1/2	cups skim milk, divided
2/3	cup long grain rice
1/4	cup sugar
1/3	cup raisins
1/2	cup egg substitute
2	tsp vanilla
1/2	tsp cinnamon
1/4	tsp nutmeg

Spray a 4-quart sauce pan with cooking spray.

Shake evaporated milk and pour into a 4-cup glass measuring cup. Add enough milk (1 1/2 cups) to measure 4 cups. Pour milk into sauce pan; heat over medium/high heat until milk comes to a boil. Stir in rice, sugar, and raisins; cover, cook over low/medium heat, stirring frequently, for 30 to 35 minutes or until rice is tender.

In the same measuring cup, mix reserved 1 cup milk, egg substitute, vanilla and spices until well blended. Raise heat to medium and stir egg mixture into cooked rice mixture, stirring constantly, until slightly thickened but still loose and creamy, about 3 minutes.

Remove from heat and pour into dessert dishes. Store leftovers, covered, in refrigerator. Can be served warm or chilled.

❖ For extra creamy rice pudding, combine 1/2 cup nonfat ricotta cheese in measuring cup along with milk, vanilla, egg whites and spices. Proceed as directed.

GLORIFIED RICE PUDDING

A NICE CHANGE FROM TRADITIONAL RICE PUDDING
Prep time: 15 min   Chill time: 4 hrs
Serves: 8   Serving size: 1/2 Cup
Exchanges: 1 Starch and 1/2 Fruit (1 Carbohydrate Choice)
Analysis per serving: 116 Calories, 22 g Carbohydrate, 3 g Protein,
2 g Fat, 53 mg Cholesterol, 126 mg Sodium, 1 g Fiber

1	**8-ounce can juice-packed crushed pineapple**
3	**Tbs sugar, divided**
4	**tsp cornstarch**
1/2	**cup skim milk**
2	**large egg yolks**
1/2	**tsp vanilla**
Pasteurized dried egg white for 2 egg whites	
Water	**(see page 13)**
1/8	**tsp cream of tartar**
1 1/2	**cups cooked brown rice**
1/4	**cup maraschino cherries or fresh cherries, chopped**

Drain pineapple juice into a 4-cup measuring cup; set drained pineapple aside. Use a whisk or a fork to stir 1 Tbs of sugar and cornstarch into juice; blend in milk. Microwave on High 4 to 6 minutes, stirring every 2 minutes, until thickened. Set aside.

In a small bowl, use same whisk or fork to beat yolks. Stir 1 Tbs of hot milk mixture into yolks. Stir blended yolks into milk mixture and microwave on Medium for 1 or 2 minutes or until thick. Stir in vanilla. Set aside.

While milk is warming, use a medium bowl to combine dried egg white, water and cream of tartar. Beat with electric mixer at high speed until foamy. Gradually beat in remaining 2 Tbs of sugar, scraping bowl occasionally; beat until stiff peaks form when lifted with a rubber spatula. Use spatula to fold meringue into pudding until no white streaks remain. Gently fold in drained pineapple, cooked rice and chopped cherries. Cover and chill about 4 hours before serving.

PINEAPPLE TAPIOCA

PINEAPPLE GIVES THIS DESSERT A TASTY TROPICAL FLAVOR
Prep time: 15 min   Cook time: 30 min
Serves: 4   Serving size: 1/4 Portion
Exchanges: 1 Skim milk and 1/2 Fruit (1 Carbohydrate Choice)
Analysis per serving: 123 Calories, 21 g Carbohydrate, 5 g Protein,
2 g Fat, 55 mg Cholesterol, 64 mg Sodium, 0 g Fiber

3	**Tbs quick cooking tapioca**
1	**Tbs sugar**
1 1/2	**cups skim milk**
1	**large egg yolk**
1	**8-ounce can juice-packed crushed pineapple**
1/2	**tsp vanilla extract**
Pasteurized dried egg white for 1 egg white	
Water	**(see page 13)**

In a 4-cup glass measuring cup, mix together tapioca, sugar, milk, and
egg yolk. Let stand for 5 minutes. Stir and microwave on High for 6
minutes, stirring every 3 minutes or until mixture boils and thickens. Stir in
undrained pineapple and vanilla.

In a medium bowl, beat dried egg white and water with electric mixer on
high speed until soft peaks form when beaters are lifted. Gently fold
beaten meringue into pudding mixture until no white streaks remain.
Spoon into 4 dessert dishes; chill about 30 minutes.

FLUFFY BLUEBERRY TAPIOCA

FOR EXTRA APPEAL SERVE IN PARFAIT GLASSES
Prep time: 20 min   Cook time: 1 hr
Serves: 8   Serving size: 1/2 Cup
Exchanges: 1/2 Skim milk, 1/2 Fruit and 1/2 Fat (1 Carbohydrate Choice)
Analysis per serving: 102 Calories, 17 g Carbohydrate, 4 g Protein,
2 g Fat, 54 mg Cholesterol, 59 mg Sodium, 1 g Fiber

3	Tbs quick-cooking tapioca
4	Tbs sugar, divided
2	large egg yolks
2 1/2	cups skim milk
1	tsp vanilla extract
1/2	tsp dried orange peel
Pasteurized dried egg white for 2 egg whites	
Water	(see page 13)
2	cups fresh blueberries, washed and drained

In a 4-cup glass measuring cup, blend tapioca, 2 Tbs sugar and egg yolks. Gradually stir in milk. Let stand for 5 minutes. Stir and microwave on High for 3 minutes. Stir and microwave every 3 minutes until mixture starts to boil and thicken. Set aside for 10 minutes to cool. Stir in vanilla and orange peel.

In a medium bowl, beat dried egg white and water with electric mixer at high speed until soft peaks form. Gradually add remaining 2 Tbs of sugar. Beat until stiff. Gently stir beaten meringue into tapioca mixture until no white streaks remain. Stir in blueberries.

Spoon into dessert dishes. Chill about 1 hour before serving.

BREAD PUDDING

A DELICIOUS DESSERT OR A GREAT BREAKFAST
Prep time: 20 min   Cook time: 45 min
Serves: 6   Serving size: 1/2 Cup
Exchanges: 1 Skim milk and 1/2 Starch (1 Carbohydrate Choice)
Analysis per serving: 148 Calories, 21 g Carbohydrate, 13 g Protein,
1 g Fat, 1 mg Cholesterol, 210 mg Sodium, 2 g Fiber

1 1/2	cups nonfat ricotta cheese
3/4	cup skim milk
1/2	cup egg substitute
2	Tbs sugar
1	tsp cinnamon
1	tsp vanilla
1	tsp butter extract
4	slices whole wheat bread, cut into 1/2-inch cubes
1/4	cup snipped dates

Spray a 1 1/2-quart casserole with cooking spray. Have 13x9x2-inch pan ready.

In a food processor or blender, whirl ricotta cheese, milk, egg substitute, sugar, cinnamon, vanilla and butter extract until smooth. Scrape sides and whirl again. Pour into the prepared casserole. Add bread cubes and dates and stir to moisten. Let stand 15 minutes. Stir again.

Preheat oven to 350°F. Set filled casserole in larger pan and place in oven. Pour boiling water into the larger pan to a depth of 1-inch. Bake for 45 minutes or until knife inserted in center comes out clean. Remove pudding from water bath. Serve warm or cold. Cover and refrigerate leftovers.

To microwave: No need for waterbath. Microwave on High for 2 minutes; rotate; microwave on Medium 8 to 10 minutes, rotating every 2 minutes until almost set. Center will be slightly soft. Let rest at least 15 minutes before serving warm. Cover leftovers and refrigerate. Prep time: 20 min Cook time: 8 min

❖ 4 slices of cinnamon raisin bread can be substituted for whole wheat bread and dates.

ORANGE SOUFFLE

AN ELEGANT ENDING TO A SPECIAL DINNER
Prep time: 10 min   Cook time: 25 min
Serves: 8   Serving size:1/8 Portion
Exchanges: 1 Skim milk (1 Carbohydrate Choice)
Analysis per serving: 71 Calories, 12 g Carbohydrate, 5 g Protein,
0 g Fat, 1 mg Cholesterol, 70 mg Sodium, 0 g Fiber

2	Tbs cornstarch
2	Tbs sugar
3/4	cup evaporated skim milk
3	Tbs orange juice concentrate, thawed
2	Tbs low-sugar orange marmalade
1	tsp vanilla
6	large egg whites, at room temperature
1/2	tsp cream of tartar

Preheat oven to 425°F. Spray a 2-quart souffle dish with cooking spray.

In a 4-cup glass measuring cup, combine cornstarch and sugar. Using a whisk or fork, stir in milk, orange juice concentrate, marmalade and vanilla. Microwave on High for 3 minutes, stir, microwave 2 minutes more or until thickened. Set aside. Let cool.

In a medium bowl, beat egg whites and cream of tartar with electric mixer at high speed until egg whites are stiff but not dry. Stir 1/4 of egg white mixture into milk mixture; fold in remaining whites until no white streaks remain.

Spoon mixture into prepared souffle dish. Bake at 425°F for 1 minute. Reduce oven to 375°F and bake 24 minutes or until puffed and golden. SERVE IMMEDIATELY. Do not open oven door during baking.

❖ Have ingredients measured in 4-cup glass measuring cup and bowl and utensils ready so that souffle can be prepared, baked and served promptly. Your guests will think you spent hours in the kitchen instead of minutes.

ORANGE HONEY CUSTARD

THIS CUSTARD IS SO SMOOTH, IT JUST SLIDES DOWN
Prep time: 10 min   Cook time: 8 min microwave or 40 min oven
Serves: 6   Serving size: 1/2 Cup
Exchanges: 1 Skim milk and 1/2 Fruit (1 Carbohydrate Choice)
Analysis per serving: 127 Calories, 15 g Carbohydrate, 10 g Protein,
3 g Fat, 107 mg Cholesterol, 131 mg Sodium, 0 g Fiber

2	cups skim milk
2	Tbs honey
1/2	cup nonfat dry milk powder
3	large eggs, beaten or 3/4 cup egg substitute
1	tsp orange juice concentrate, thawed
1/2	tsp dried orange peel or grated fresh orange peel

Spray a 1-quart casserole with cooking spray.

In a 4-cup glass measuring cup, microwave milk on High for 3 minutes; stir and cook an additional 3 or 4 minutes or until milk is scalded. Use a whisk to stir in honey and dry milk powder until smooth; set aside to cool.

In a small bowl, use same whisk to combine eggs, orange juice concentrate and orange peel. Slowly add to milk mixture, stirring to thoroughly combine.

Pour into the prepared casserole. Place filled casserole into a larger casserole filled with 1/2-inch of hot water. Place both casseroles on turntable in microwave. Cook on Medium for 7 to 12 minutes or until slightly firm but still soft in center. Let rest 30 minutes before serving. May be served at room temperature or chilled. Refrigerate covered leftovers. (If turntable is not available, be sure to rotate filled casseroles every 2 minutes to ensure even cooking.)

❖ Custard may also be baked. Pour mixture into prepared casserole. Place filled casserole in a 13x9x2-inch pan; set pan on rack in preheated 350°F oven. Fill larger pan with 1 inch of hot water. Bake custard for 40 to 50 minutes or until knife inserted in center comes out clean. Cool custard at least 15 minutes before serving. Refrigerate covered leftovers.

SIMPLE VANILLA PUDDING

A SNAP TO MAKE — SERVE WITH FRUIT OR USE AS A PIE FILLING
Prep time: 10 min   Cook time: 1 hr
Serves: 4   Serving size: 1/2 Cup
Exchanges: 1 Skim milk (1 Carbohydrate Choice)
Analysis per serving: 90 Calories, 18 g Carbohydrate, 4 g Protein,
0 g Fat, 2 mg Cholesterol, 64 mg Sodium, 0 g Fiber

2	**cups skim milk, divided**
2	**Tbs sugar**
3	**Tbs cornstarch**
2	**tsp vanilla extract**

In a 4-cup measuring cup, measure 1 1/2 cups milk. Microwave on High for 3 to 4 minutes or until milk is scalded.

Meanwhile, in small bowl combine sugar and cornstarch. Use a small whisk or fork to stir in remaining 1/2 cup milk. Mix until smooth. Stir mixture into scalded milk until well blended. Return to microwave and cook on High for 1 1/2 to 2 minutes or until thickened.

Let mixture rest for 1 minute, then stir in vanilla. Spoon into 4 dessert dishes or let cool about 10 minutes and combine with fruit before spooning into dishes or a baked pie crust. Chill at least one hour or until pudding is firm before serving.

❖ This recipe makes an excellent pie. See page 177 for BANANA CREAM TART.

Quick or Tea Breads

Quick breads are aptly named — they are quick and simple to prepare. These breads may be simple to prepare but do take at least 45 minutes to bake. Some must be baked for over an hour.

Quick breads are also called tea breads since they are the perfect accompaniment to hot or iced tea or coffee. They are delicious for breakfast along with an egg or yogurt or spread with yogurt cheese, nonfat cream cheese, even natural peanut butter and low-sugar jams and jellies.

Tea breads add a special touch to lunch when used as a sandwich bread or as an addition to salad or soup. Quick breads make terrific snacks since a slice is filling and low in fat and sugar. When served with fresh fruit, a slice of tea bread is a tasty finale to a meal. Many tea or quick breads taste even more delicious when sliced and toasted.

Some quick breads contain fruit for added sweetness and fiber. Many also contain chopped nuts which have been toasted. It is not required to toast nuts before adding to the batter, although toasted nuts add more flavor. Therefore, the amount of nuts called for in many recipes can be reduced which also lowers the fat content. Cool toasted nuts slightly before stirring into batter. When following recipes in this book, there is no need to reduce the amount of nuts.

Similar to muffins, coffee cakes and scones, do NOT overmix quick or tea breads. Combine dry ingredients and stir in fruit and/or nuts. Mix wet ingredients separately from dry ingredients and then combine both dry and wet ingredients just until moistened. Spoon into prepared pan(s) and use a rubber spatula to spread batter evenly; bake as directed.

If you are baking more than one loaf on the same oven rack, be sure that there is at least two inches between baking pans so that the breads bake evenly. Ovens vary; therefore, it is recommended that you test the bread before removing from the oven. Insert a pick in the center of the baked loaf. If the pick comes out clean, the bread is done. If there is some batter on the pick, bake another 5 to 10 minutes or until the pick comes out clean. Place baked breads on a rack and cool about 10 minutes. Loosen bread in pan with a knife and remove bread from pan. Serve or cool completely and store wrapped in plastic wrap or aluminum foil or in a plastic bag. Quick or tea breads can be frozen up to 3 months.

Many quick or tea breads will be easier to slice if stored, covered, for at least 4 hours or overnight. I recommend using a serrated knife to slice the breads.

Many quick breads develop a crack in the center. This is typical. If the bread contains some sort of fruit, do not keep at room temperature more than two days or it can become rancid. Store in the refrigerator. When ready to serve, slice and toast or slice and place on a paper plate and microwave until warm.

If you prefer to bake small loaves instead of one large loaf, three small loaf pans, 2x5-inches, can be substituted for a 9x5-inch loaf pan. Or, one 3x7-inch and one 3x5-inch can be substituted for a 9x5-inch loaf pan. If glass or Pyrex loaf pan(s) are used, lower oven temperature by 25°.

As with most of my baked goods recipes, I have used whole-wheat flour and all-purpose flour. If you prefer to use only all-purpose flour, do so. I prefer using a mixture of both since many vitamins and minerals are removed in milling white flour and whole-wheat flour has natural fiber.

Be sure to read each recipe before starting so that you have all ingredients and utensils available before you begin. I recommend that you read the entire recipe before spooning the batter into the baking pan(s) so that you are certain that all ingredients have been included and directions have been followed.

APRICOT BREAD

THE APRICOT FLAVOR IS SUBTLE AND THE TEXTURE CHEWY
Prep time: 10 min   Bake time: 60 min
Makes: 1 9x5-inch Loaf   Serving size: 1 Slice, 1/16 Portion
Exchanges:1/2 Starch, 1/2 Fruit and 1/2 Fat (1 Carbohydrate Choice)
Analysis per serving: 101 Calories, 18 g Carbohydrate, 3 g Protein,
2 g Fat, 13 mg Cholesterol, 108 mg Sodium, 2 g Fiber

1/4	chopped pecans or walnuts (optional)
1	cup whole-wheat flour
1	cup all-purpose flour
2	tsp baking powder
1/4	tsp baking soda
1/4	tsp salt
1/4	cup sugar
1	tsp dried orange peel or grated fresh orange peel
1/2	cup chopped dried apricots
2	Tbs olive or canola oil
1	large egg or 1/4 cup egg substitute
3/4	cup orange juice

Preheat oven 350°F. If using nuts, place nuts on baking sheet and toast 3 to 5 minutes or until toasted; set aside. Spray 9x5-inch loaf pan with cooking spray.

Sift flours, baking powder, baking soda, salt and sugar into a large bowl. If grains remain in sifter, stir into dry ingredients. Stir in orange peel, chopped apricots and nuts, if using.

In small bowl, use a whisk or a fork to combine oil, egg and orange juice. Add wet ingredients to dry ingredients and combine just until moistened. Spoon into prepared pan. Bake 60 to 65 minutes or until a pick inserted in center comes out clean. Cool on rack for 10 minutes. Loosen bread from pan with a knife and remove to rack to cool. Store covered up to 2 days at room temperature or freeze up to 3 months.

Bread will be easier to slice if covered and left to stand at least 4 hours or overnight.

❖ Snip apricots into small pieces with scissors. Spray scissors with cooking spray so that apricots do not stick.

APPLE OATMEAL LOAF

AN APPEALING BREAD WITH A TOUCH OF SPICE AND CHUNKY APPLES
Prep time: 10 min   Bake time: 60 min
Makes: 1 5x8-inch Loaf   Serving size: 1 Slice, 1/16 Portion
Exchanges: 1 Starch and 1/2 Fat (1 Carbohydrate Choice)
Analysis per serving: 107 Calories, 16 g Carbohydrate, 3 g Protein,
4 g Fat, 0 mg Cholesterol, 172 mg Sodium, 2 g Fiber

1/4	chopped walnuts (optional)
3/4	cup whole-wheat flour
3/4	cup all-purpose flour
2	tsp baking powder
1	tsp baking soda
1/4	tsp salt
1	tsp cinnamon
1/2	tsp nutmeg
1/4	cup brown sugar
1	cup old-fashioned oats
1 1/2	cups diced, peeled apple (1 large)
1/2	cup egg substitute
1/4	cup olive or canola oil
1/4	cup skim milk
1	Tbs lemon juice

Preheat oven 350°F. If using nuts, place on baking sheet and bake 3 to 5 minutes or until toasted; set aside. Spray 5x8-inch loaf pan.

Sift flours, baking powder, baking soda, salt, cinnamon and nutmeg into a large bowl. If grains remain in sifter, stir into dry ingredients. Stir in brown sugar, oats, diced apples and nuts, if using, until well blended.

In a glass measuring cup or small bowl use a whisk or a fork to combine egg substitute, oil, milk and lemon juice. Pour wet ingredients into dry ingredients and mix just until blended. Do not over mix.

Spoon into prepared pan. Bake 60 to 65 minutes or until pick inserted in center comes out clean. Cool on rack 10 minutes. Loosen bread from pan with a knife and remove to rack to cool. Store covered.

Loaf will be easier to slice if left covered at room temperature for at least 4 hours or overnight. May be frozen up to 3 months. Do not leave at room temperature more than 2 days.

APPLESAUCE BREAD

APPLESAUCE ADDS NATURAL SWEETNESS, TEXTURE AND FLAVOR
Prep time: 10 min   Bake time: 45 min
Makes: 1 9x5-inch loaf   Serving size: 1 Slice, 1/16 Portion
Exchanges: 1 Starch (1 Carbohydrate Choice)
Analysis per serving: 94 Calories, 18 g Carbohydrate, 3 g Protein,
1 g Fat, 0 mg Cholesterol, 64 mg Sodium, 2 g Fiber

1/4	cup chopped nuts
1	cup whole-wheat flour
1	cup all-purpose flour
1	tsp baking powder
1/2	tsp baking soda
1/4	tsp salt
1 1/2	cups unsweetened applesauce
1/4	cup honey
2	large egg whites

Preheat oven 350°F. Place nuts on baking sheet and bake 3 to 5 minutes or until toasted; set aside. Spray 9x5-inch loaf pan with cooking spray.

In a large bowl, combine flours, baking powder, baking soda, salt and toasted nuts. In small bowl, use a whisk or a fork to combine applesauce, honey and egg whites until well mixed. Stir applesauce mixture into dry ingredients just until moistened; do not over mix.

Spoon in prepared pan. Bake 45 to 50 minutes or until pick inserted in center comes out clean. Cool 10 minutes. Use a knife to loosen bread; remove from pan. Cool.

Store, covered, at least 4 hours or overnight for easier slicing. Refrigerate after 2 days. Can be frozen up to 3 months. Delicious sliced and toasted.

BANANA NUT BREAD

A FAVORITE QUICK BREAD — SO SWEET AND TASTY
Prep time: 10 min   Bake time: 60 min
Makes: 1 9x5-inch Loaf   Serving size: 1 Slice, 1/16 Portion
Exchanges: 1 Starch, 1/2 Fruit and 1 Fat (2 Carbohydrate Choices)
Analysis per serving: 143 Calories, 23 g Carbohydrate, 3 g Protein,
5 g Fat, 13 mg Cholesterol, 125 mg Sodium, 2 g Fiber

1/4	cup chopped pecans or walnuts
1	cup whole-wheat flour
1	cup all-purpose flour
2	tsp baking powder
1/2	tsp baking soda
1/4	tsp salt
1/2	tsp nutmeg
1/4	cup sugar
1 1/2	cups mashed ripe bananas (3 medium or 2 large)
1/4	cup olive or canola oil
2	Tbs orange juice
1	large egg or 1/4 cup egg substitute
1/2	tsp vanilla extract

Preheat oven 350°F. Place nuts on baking sheet and bake 3 to 5 minutes or until toasted; set aside. Spray 9x5-inch loaf pan with cooking spray.

In large bowl, combine flours, baking powder, baking soda, salt, nutmeg, sugar and nuts.

In a small bowl use a whisk or a fork to combine mashed banana, oil, orange juice, egg and vanilla until well blended. Stir wet ingredients into dry ingredients and mix until well blended.

Spoon into prepared pan and bake 60 to 65 minutes or until pick inserted in center comes out clean. Cool on rack for 10 minutes. Use a knife to loosen bread from pan and remove to rack to cool.

When cool, store covered at least 4 hours or overnight for easier slicing. Do not leave at room temperature for more than 2 days; refrigerate. Can be frozen up to 3 months.

MINI BLUEBERRY LOAVES

BURSTING WITH THE ENTICING FLAVOR OF BLUEBERRIES
Prep time: 5 min   Bake time: 50 min
Makes: 3 Mini loaves   Serving size: 1 Slice, 1/15 Portion
Exchanges: 1 Starch and 1/2 Fruit (2 Carbohydrate Choices)
Analysis per serving: 117 Calories, 23 g Carbohydrate, 4 g Protein,
1 g Fat, 0 mg Cholesterol, 172 mg Sodium, 3 g Fiber

1 1/2	**cups whole-wheat flour**
1 1/2	**cups all-purpose flour**
1	**Tbs baking powder**
1/2	**tsp baking soda**
1/4	**tsp salt**
1/2	**tsp nutmeg**
1	**tsp dried lemon peel or grated fresh lemon peel**
2	**cups fresh or frozen blueberries**
1	**Tbs olive or canola oil**
1/2	**cup egg substitute**
1	**cup unsweetened applesauce**

Preheat oven 350°F. Spray 3 mini loaf pans (2x5-inch) with cooking spray.

In a large bowl, combine flours, baking powder, baking soda, salt, nutmeg and lemon peel until well mixed. Stir in blueberries until coated with flour mixture.

In a small bowl, use a whisk or a fork to combine oil, egg substitute and applesauce until well blended. Stir wet ingredients into dry ingredients until blended; do not over mix.

Spoon into prepared pans. Bake 40 to 45 minutes or until pick inserted in center of breads comes out clean. Cool in pan on rack for 10 minutes. Loosen loaves with a knife; remove from pans and cool on rack.

When cool, store covered at least 4 hours or overnight for easier slicing. May be frozen up to 3 months. Refrigerate after 2 days at room temperature.

❖ Can also be baked in a 9x5-inch loaf pan which has been sprayed with cooking spray. Bake 55 to 60 minutes or until pick inserted in center comes out clean. Proceed as directed.

TEMPTING BLUEBERRY BREAD

BRAN IS ADDED FOR EXTRA FIBER
Prep time: 10 min   Bake time: 50 min
Makes: 1 9x5-inch Loaf   Serving size: 1 Slice, 1/16 Portion
Exchanges: 1/2 Starch, 1/2 Fruit and 1/2 Fat (1 Carbohydrate Choice)
Analysis per serving: 90 Calories, 16 g Carbohydrate, 2 g Protein,
2 g Fat, 13 mg Cholesterol, 127 mg Sodium, 2 g Fiber

1/4	cup chopped nuts (optional)
1/2	cup bran
1	cup all-purpose flour
3/4	cup whole-wheat flour
2	tsp baking powder
1/2	tsp baking soda
1/4	tsp salt
1/2	tsp nutmeg
2	tsp dried lemon peel or grated fresh lemon peel
1/4	cup brown sugar
1	cup fresh or frozen blueberries
3/4	cup orange juice
2	Tbs olive or canola oil
1	large egg or 1/4 cup egg substitute

Preheat oven 350°F. If using nuts, place on baking sheet and bake 3 to 5 minutes or until toasted; set aside. Spray 9x5-inch loaf pan with cooking spray.

In large bowl, combine bran, flours, baking powder, baking soda, salt, nutmeg, lemon peel and brown sugar until well blended. Stir in blueberries and nuts, if using, until berries are coated with flour mixture.

In small bowl, use a whisk or a fork to combine orange juice, oil and egg until well mixed. Stir wet ingredients into dry ingredients until blended; do not over mix.

Spoon into prepared pan and bake 50 to 55 minutes or until pick inserted in center comes out clean. Cool on rack for 10 minutes. Loosen bread with a knife and remove from pan; cool on rack.

When cool, cover, and store at least 4 hours or overnight before slicing. After 2 days, refrigerate. Can be frozen up to 3 months.

QUICK BRAN BREAD

MOLASSES ADDS A RICH MELLOW FLAVOR
Prep time: 10 min   Bake time: 50 min
Makes: 1 9x5-inch Loaf   Serving size: 1 Slice, 1/16 Portion
Exchanges: 1/2 Starch, 1/2 Fruit and 1 Fat (1 Carbohydrate Choice)
Analysis per serving: 122 Calories, 20 g Carbohydrate, 4 g Protein,
4 g Fat, 14 mg Cholesterol, 167 mg Sodium, 3 g Fiber

1/4	cup chopped walnuts (optional)
1 1/2	cups skim milk
1/4	cup molasses
1	cup bran
1	cup whole-wheat flour
1	cup all-purpose flour
3	tsp baking powder
1/2	tsp baking soda
1/4	tsp salt
2	Tbs sugar
1/4	cup olive or canola oil
1	large egg or 1/4 cup egg substitute

Preheat oven 350°F. If using nuts, place on baking sheet and bake 3 to 5 minutes or until toasted; set aside. Spray 9x5-inch loaf pan.

In small bowl, mix milk, molasses and bran; let stand 5 minutes or until bran is soft. Stir and set aside. In large bowl, combine flours, baking powder, baking soda, salt and sugar; stir in nuts, if using.

Use a whisk or a fork to mix oil and egg into bran mixture until well blended. Stir wet ingredients into dry ingredients and mix just until moistened. Do not over mix.

Spoon into prepared pan. Bake 50 to 55 minutes or until pick inserted in center comes out clean. Cool on rack for 10 minutes. Use a knife to loosen bread and remove from pan. Cool on rack.

Store, covered, at least 4 hours or overnight for easier slicing. Can be frozen up to 3 months.

SPICY CARROT BREAD

A YUMMY CHUNKY TEA BREAD
Prep time: 10 min   Bake time: 45 min
Makes: 1 5x8-inch Loaf   Serving size: 1 Slice, 1/16 Portion
Exchanges: 1 Starch and 1/2 Fat (1 Carbohydrate Choice)
Analysis per serving: 97 Calories, 13 g Carbohydrate, 2 g Protein,
4 g Fat, 13 mg Cholesterol, 132 mg Sodium, 1 g Fiber

1	cup whole-wheat flour
1/2	cup all-purpose flour
2	tsp baking powder
1/2	tsp baking soda
1/4	tsp salt
1	tsp cinnamon
1/4	tsp ginger
1	tsp dried orange peel or grated fresh orange peel
1/4	cup brown sugar
1 1/2	cups shredded carrots
2	Tbs golden raisins
1	Tbs chopped walnuts
1/4	cup olive or canola oil
1/3	cup skim milk
2	Tbs orange juice
1	large egg or 1/4 cup egg substitute
1	tsp vanilla

Preheat oven 375°F. Spray 5x8-inch loaf pan with cooking spray.

In large bowl, combine flours, baking powder, baking soda, salt, cinnamon, ginger, orange peel and brown sugar until well mixed. Stir in carrots, raisins and nuts.

In small bowl, use a whisk or a fork to combine oil, milk, orange juice, egg and vanilla until well blended. Stir wet ingredients into dry ingredients until moistened; do not over mix.

Spoon batter into prepared pan. Bake 45 to 50 minutes or until pick inserted in center comes out clean. Cool on rack for 10 minutes. Use a knife to loosen bread; remove from pan. Cool.

Store, covered, at least 4 hours or overnight for easier slicing. Refrigerate after 2 days. Can be frozen up to 3 months.

CHOCOLICIOUS QUICK BREAD

A CHOCOLATE LOVER'S DELIGHT
Prep time: 10 min   Bake time: 55 min
Makes: 1 9x5-inch Loaf   Serving size: 1 Slice, 1/16 Portion
Exchanges: 1 Starch, 1/2 Fruit and 1 Fat (1 Carbohydrate Choice)
Analysis per serving: 132 Calories, 21 g Carbohydrate, 4 g Protein,
4 g Fat, 14 mg Cholesterol, 127 mg Sodium, 2 g Fiber

1 1/4	cups whole-wheat flour
1 1/4	cups all-purpose flour
3	tsp baking powder
1/4	tsp salt
1/4	cup cocoa
1/3	cup sugar
1	large egg or 1/4 cup egg substitute
1 1/3	cups skim milk
2	Tbs orange juice
1/4	cup olive or canola oil
1	Tbs chopped nuts

Preheat oven 350°F. Spray 9x5-inch loaf pan with cooking spray.

Sift flours, baking powder, salt, cocoa and sugar in a large bowl. If grains remain in sifter, stir into dry ingredients.

In small bowl, use a whisk or a fork to combine egg, milk, orange juice and oil until well blended. Stir wet ingredients into dry ingredients just until moistened; do not over mix.

Spoon batter into prepared pan. Sprinkle with nuts and press nuts into bread. Bake 55 to 60 minutes or until pick inserted in center comes out clean. Cool on rack for 10 minutes. Use a knife to loosen bread and remove from pan. Cool.

Store, covered, at least 4 hours or overnight for easier slicing. Can be frozen up to 3 months.

CRANBERRY NUT BREAD

A TOPNOTCH TEA BREAD FOR BREAKFAST, LUNCH OR DINNER
Prep time: 10 min   Bake time: 55 min
Makes: 1 9x5-inch Loaf   Serving size: 1 Slice, 1/16 Portion
Exchanges: 1 Starch, 1/2 Fruit and 1 Fat (1 Carbohydrate Choice)
Analysis per serving: 132 Calories, 17 g Carbohydrate, 3 g Protein,
6 g Fat, 13 mg Cholesterol, 148 mg Sodium, 2 g Fiber

1/2	cup chopped nuts
1	cup whole-wheat flour
1	cup all-purpose flour
1 1/2	tsp baking powder
1	tsp baking soda
1/4	tsp salt
1	Tbs dried orange peel or grated fresh orange peel
1/4	cup sugar
1	cup cranberries
1/4	cup olive or canola oil
3/4	cup orange juice
1	large egg or 1/4 cup egg substitute

Preheat oven 350°F. Place nuts on baking sheet and bake 3 to 5 minutes or until toasted; set aside. Spray 9x5-inch loaf pan with cooking spray.

Sift flours, baking powder, baking soda and salt into a large bowl. If grains remain in sifter, just add to flour mixture. Stir in peel, sugar, cranberries and toasted nuts until well mixed.

In a small bowl, use a whisk or a fork to combine oil, orange juice and egg until well blended. Stir wet ingredients into dry ingredients just until blended; do not over mix.

Spoon batter into prepared pan. Bake 55 to 60 minutes or until pick inserted in center comes out clean. Cool on rack for 10 minutes. Use a knife to loosen bread and remove from pan. Cool.

Store, covered, at least 4 hours or overnight for easier slicing. Refrigerate after 2 days. Can be frozen up to 3 months.

DATE NUT BREAD

USE NONFAT CREAM CHEESE OR YOGURT CHEESE (page 83) AS A SPREAD
Prep time: 10 min   Bake time: 60 min
Makes: 1 9x5-inch Loaf   Serving size: 1 Slice, 1/16 Portion
Exchanges: 1 1/2 Starch and 1 Fat (2 Carbohydrate Choices)
Analysis per serving: 175 Calories, 28 g Carbohydrate, 4 g Protein,
5 g Fat, 13 mg Cholesterol, 334 mg Sodium, 3 g Fiber

1/2	cup chopped pecans
1 1/2	cups skim milk
3/4	cup chopped dates
1 1/2	cups whole-wheat flour
1 1/2	cups all-purpose flour
1/4	cup sugar
3	tsp baking powder
1/2	tsp baking soda
1/4	tsp salt
3	Tbs olive or canola oil
3	Tbs orange juice
1	large egg or 1/4 cup egg substitute
1	tsp vanilla

Preheat oven 350°F. Place nuts on baking sheet and bake 3 to 5 minutes or until toasted; set aside. Spray 9x5-inch loaf pan.

Microwave milk in a 4-cup glass measuring cup on High for 4 minutes. Stir in dates; cool.

Sift flours, sugar, baking powder, baking soda and salt into a large bowl. If grains remain in sifter, stir into dry ingredients. Stir in toasted nuts.

Add oil, juice, egg and vanilla to cooled milk and use a fork to combine until well mixed. Add wet ingredients to dry ingredients and mix until blended. Do not overmix.

Spoon in prepared pan. Let rest 20 minutes.

Bake 60 to 70 minutes or until pick inserted in center comes out clean. Cool on rack for 10 minutes. Use a knife to loosen bread and remove from pan; cool.

Store, covered, at least 4 hours or overnight for easier slicing. Can be frozen up to 3 months.

PEANUT BUTTER BREAD

A TASTY WHOLESOME BREAD
Prep time: 10 min   Bake time: 45 min
Makes: 1 9x5-inch Loaf   Serving size: 1 Slice, 1/16 Portion
Exchanges: 1/2 Lean meat, 1 Starch, 1/2 Fruit and 1 Fat (1 Carbohydrate Choice)
Analysis per serving: 165 Calories, 22 g Carbohydrate, 6 g Protein,
6 g Fat, 0 mg Cholesterol, 138 mg Sodium, 2 g Fiber

1	cup whole-wheat flour
1	cup all-purpose flour
1	cup old-fashioned oats
1	Tbs baking powder
1/4	tsp salt
1 1/2	cups skim milk
2	Tbs olive or canola oil
1/2	cup natural chunky peanut butter
1/4	cup honey
1/2	cup egg substitute
1/2	cup raisins (optional)

Preheat oven 350°F. Spray 9x5-inch loaf pan with cooking spray.

In large bowl, combine flours, oats, baking powder and salt.

In a small bowl, use a whisk or a fork to combine milk, oil, peanut butter, honey and egg substitute until well blended. Add wet ingredients to dry ingredients and stir just to moisten; do not over mix. If desired, stir in raisins.

Spoon into prepared pan. Bake 40 to 45 minutes or until pick inserted in center comes out clean. Cool on rack for 10 minutes. Use a knife to loosen bread; remove bread from pan. Cool.

Store, covered, at least 4 hours or overnight for easier slicing. Can be frozen up to 3 months.

POPPY SEED BREAD

SERVE WARM OR TOASTED WITH YOUR FAVORITE JAM — SUPERB!
Prep time: 10 min   Bake time: 40 min
Makes: 2 3x7-inch Loaves   Serving size: 1 Slice, 1/24 Portion
Exchanges: 1 Starch and 1/2 Fat (1 Carbohydrate Choice)
Analysis per serving: 113 Calories, 17 g Carbohydrate, 3 g Protein,
3 g Fat, 0 mg Cholesterol, 89 mg Sodium, 1 g Fiber

2	cups all-purpose flour
1 1/2	cups whole-wheat flour
4	tsp baking powder
1	Tbs poppy seed
1	tsp dried lemon peel or grated fresh lemon peel
3/4	cup egg substitute
1 1/4	cups skim milk
1/4	cup olive or canola oil
1/4	cup honey

Preheat oven 350°F. Spray two 3x7-inch loaf pans with cooking spray.

In large bowl, combine flours, baking powder, poppy seed and lemon peel.

In small bowl, use a whisk or a fork to combine egg substitute, milk, oil and honey until well blended. Stir wet ingredients into dry ingredients just until moistened; do not over mix.

Spoon batter into prepared pans. Bake 40 to 45 minutes or until pick inserted in center comes out clean. Cool on rack for 10 minutes. Use a knife to loosen bread; remove from pan. Serve warm.

Store covered. Can be frozen up to 3 months. Delicious sliced and toasted or reheated on paper towel or paper plate in microwave until warm.

PINEAPPLE BREAD

A QUICK FIX BREAD THAT IS A REAL TUMMY PLEASER
Prep time: 10 min   Bake time: 60 min
Makes: 1 9x5-inch Loaf   Serving size: 1 Slice, 1/16 Portioin
Exchanges: 1/2 Starch, 1/2 Fruit and 1/2 Fat (1 Carbohydrate Choice)
Analysis per serving: 94 Calories, 16 g Carbohydrate, 2 g Protein,
2 g Fat, 13 mg Cholesterol, 134 mg Sodium, 1 g Fiber

1/4	cup chopped nuts (optional)
1	cup whole-wheat flour
1	cup all-purpose flour
1	tsp baking powder
1	tsp baking soda
1/4	tsp salt
1/4	cup sugar
1	large egg or 1/4 cup egg substitute
2	Tbs olive or canola oil
3/4	tsp vanilla
1	8-ounce can juice-packed crushed pineapple, undrained

Preheat oven 350°F. If using nuts, place on baking sheet and bake 3 to 5 minutes or until toasted; set aside. Spray 9x5-inch loaf pan with cooking spray.

Sift flours, baking powder, baking soda, salt and sugar into a large bowl. If grains remain in sifter, stir into dry ingredients. Stir in toasted nuts if using.

In small bowl, use a fork or a whisk to combine egg, oil, vanilla and undrained pineapple until well mixed. Stir wet ingredients into dry ingredients just until blended; do not over mix.

Spoon batter into prepared pan. Bake 60 to 65 minutes or until pick inserted in center comes out clean. Cool on rack for 10 minutes. Use a knife to loosen bread; remove from pan; cool.

Store, covered, at least 4 hours or overnight for easier slicing. After 2 days, refrigerate or freeze up to 3 months.

PUMPKIN DATE BREAD

RAISINS CAN BE SUBSTITUTED FOR DATES
Prep time: 10 min   Bake time: 60 min
Makes: 1 9x5-inch Loaf   Serving size: 1 Slice, 1/16 Portion
Exchanges: 1 Starch and 1/2 Fat (1 Carbohydrate Choice)
Analysis per serving: 109 Calories, 17 g Carbohydrate, 3 g Protein,
4 g Fat, 0 mg Cholesterol, 145 mg Sodium, 2 g Fiber

1/4	cup chopped nuts (optional)
1	cup whole-wheat flour
1	cup all-purpose flour
1	tsp baking powder
1	tsp baking soda
1/4	tsp salt
1	tsp cinnamon
1/2	tsp nutmeg
1/4	tsp cloves
1/4	tsp allspice
2	Tbs brown sugar
1/3	cup chopped dates
1/2	cup egg substitute
1/4	cup olive or canola oil
1	cup canned pumpkin (NOT pie filling)
1/2	cup orange juice

Preheat oven 350°F. If using nuts, place on baking sheet and bake 3 to 5 minutes or until toasted; set aside. Spray 9x5-inch loaf pan.

In large bowl, combine flours, baking powder, baking soda, salt, cinnamon, nutmeg, cloves, allspice, brown sugar and nuts, if using. Stir in dates until coated with flour mixture.

In small bowl, use a whisk or a fork to combine egg substitute, oil, pumpkin and orange juice until well blended.

Make a well in dry ingredients. Add wet ingredients to well and mix just until blended; do not over mix.

Spoon in prepared pan. Bake 60 to 65 minutes or until pick inserted in center comes out clean. Cool on rack for 10 minutes. Use a knife to loosen bread and cool on rack.

Store, covered, at least 4 hours or overnight for easier slicing. After 2 days, refrigerate or freeze up to 3 months.

RAISIN BEER BREAD

AN UNUSUAL AND SPICY TEA BREAD
Prep time: 10 min   Bake time: 45 min
Makes: 1 9x5-inch Loaf   Serving size: 1 Slice, 1/16 Portion
Exchanges: 1 Starch and 1/2 Fruit (1 Carbohydrate Choice)
Analysis per serving: 105 Calories, 22 g Carbohydrate, 3 g Protein,
0 g Fat, 0 mg Cholesterol, 167 mg Sodium, 2 g Fiber

1 1/2	cups whole-wheat flour
1 1/2	cups all-purpose flour
2 1/2	tsp baking powder
1 1/2	tsp baking soda
1	tsp cinnamon
1/2	tsp nutmeg
1/8	tsp ground cloves
1/2	cup raisins
1	12-ounce can light beer
1	Tbs honey

Preheat oven 350°F. Spray 9x5-inch loaf pan with cooking spray.

In large bowl, combine flours, baking powder, baking soda, cinnamon,
nutmeg, cloves and raisins. Stir in beer and honey; do not over mix.

Spoon in prepared pan. Bake 45 to 50 minutes or until pick inserted in
center comes out clean. Cool on rack 10 minutes. Use a knife to loosen
bread; remove from pan. Cool.

Store covered. Can be frozen up to 3 months.

RASPBERRY BREAD

A STUPENDOUS ACCOMPANIMENT TO TEA OR COFFEE
Prep time: 10 min   Bake time: 60 min
Makes: 1 9x5-inch Loaf   Serving size: 1 Slice, 1/16 Portion
Exchanges: 1 Starch and 1/2 Fat (1 Carbohydrate Choice)
Analysis per serving: 106 Calories, 18 g Carbohydrate, 2 g Protein,
3 g Fat, 13 mg Cholesterol, 138 mg Sodium, 2 g Fiber

1/4	cup chopped nuts (optional)
1	cup whole-wheat flour
1	cup all-purpose flour
2 1/2	tsp baking powder
1/2	tsp baking soda
1/4	tsp salt
1/4	cup sugar
1	Tbs dried orange peel or grated fresh orange peel
2	cups fresh or frozen raspberries
3	Tbs olive or canola oil
1	large egg or 1/4 cup egg substitute
3/4	cup orange juice

Preheat oven 350°F. If using nuts, place on baking sheet and bake 3 to 5 minutes or until toasted; set aside. Spray 9x5-inch loaf pan with cooking spray.

Sift flours, baking powder, baking soda, salt and sugar in a large bowl. If grains remain in sifter, stir into dry ingredients. Stir in orange peel, toasted nuts, if using, and raspberries until raspberries are coated with flour.

In small bowl, using a whisk or a fork, combine oil, egg and orange juice. Gently stir wet ingredients into dry ingredients just until blended; do not over mix.

Spoon batter into prepared pan. Bake 60 to 65 minutes or until pick inserted in center comes out clean. Cool on rack for 10 minutes. Use a knife to loosen bread; remove from pan.

Store, covered, at least 4 hours or overnight for easier slicing. Refrigerate after 2 days. Can be frozen up to 3 months.

❖ 1 cup sliced strawberries can be used in place of raspberries.

SESAME TEA BREAD

TOASTING THIS BREAD MAKES IT EVEN MORE TASTY
Prep time: 10 min   Bake time: 60 min
Makes: 1 9x5-inch Loaf   Serving size: 1 Slice, 1/16 Portion
Exchanges: 1 1/2 Starch and 1 Fat (1 Carbohydrate Choice)
Analysis per serving: 150 Calories, 22 g Carbohydrate, 4 g Protein,
5 g Fat, 0 mg Cholesterol, 95 mg Sodium, 2 g Fiber

1/2	cup sesame seeds, toasted
1 1/2	cups whole-wheat flour
1 1/2	cups all-purpose flour
1	Tbs baking powder
1/4	cup sugar
1	tsp dried lemon peel or grated fresh lemon peel
1/2	cup egg substitute
1 1/2	cups skim milk
1/4	cup olive or canola oil
1	Tbs sesame seeds, untoasted

Preheat oven 350°F. Place 1/2 cup sesame seeds on baking sheet and bake 3 to 5 minutes or until toasted; set aside. Spray 9x5-inch loaf pan with cooking spray.

In large bowl, combine flours, baking powder, sugar, lemon peel and toasted sesame seeds.

In small bowl, use a whisk or a fork to combine egg substitute, milk and olive oil until well blended. Add wet ingredients to dry ingredients and combine just to moisten; do not over mix.

Spoon batter into prepared pan. Sprinkle with untoasted sesame seeds. Bake 60 to 65 minutes or until pick inserted in center comes out clean. Cool on rack for 10 minutes. Use a knife to loosen bread; remove from pan.

Tastes best served warm. Store covered.

❖ Slice and toast this bread before making scrumptious sandwiches. Absolutely wonderful!

SODA BREAD

1 1/2	cups whole-wheat flour
1 1/2	cups all-purpose flour
1/2	tsp baking powder
1	tsp baking soda
1/4	tsp salt
1/2	cup raisins
2	Tbs caraway seeds (optional)
1	large egg or 1/4 cup egg substitute
1	Tbs olive or canola oil
1	cup buttermilk

Preheat oven 350°F. Spray baking sheet with cooking spray.

In large bowl, combine flours, baking powder, baking soda, salt, raisins and caraway seeds, if using,

In small bowl, combine egg, oil and buttermilk until well mixed. Add wet ingredients to dry ingredients and mix well. Batter is very sticky.

Place dough on a floured board, sprinkle with flour and knead two or three times. Mold into a round loaf and place on prepared baking sheet. Flatten to an 8-inch circle about 1 1/2 inches thick. Using a sharp knife, mark a 1/2-inch deep cross in top of bread.

Bake 55 to 60 minutes or until pick inserted in center comes out clean. Serve at once or let cool; slice and toast.

WHOLE-WHEAT RAISIN BREAD

WHOLE-WHEAT GOODNESS IN EVERY BITE
Prep time: 10 min   Bake time: 50 min
Makes: 1 5x8-inch Loaf   Serving size: 1 Slice, 1/14 Portion
Exchanges: 1 Starch, 1/2 Fruit and 1 Fat (2 Carbohydrate Choices)
Analysis per serving: 148 Calories, 23 g Carbohydrate, 3 g Protein,
6 g Fat, 0 mg Cholesterol, 117 mg Sodium, 3 g Fiber

1/4	cup chopped walnuts
2	cups whole-wheat flour
1	tsp baking powder
1	tsp baking soda
1/2	cup raisins
2	large egg whites
1 3/4	cups buttermilk
1/4	cup olive or canola oil
1/4	cup honey

Preheat oven 375°F. Place nuts on baking sheet and bake 3 to 5 minutes or until toasted; set aside. Spray 5x8-inch loaf pan with cooking spray.

In large bowl, combine flour, baking powder, baking soda, raisins and toasted nuts.

In small bowl, use a whisk or a fork to combine egg whites, buttermilk, oil and honey until well blended. Add wet ingredients to dry ingredients and mix just until blended; do not over mix.

Spoon into prepared pan. Bake 50 to 55 minutes or until pick inserted in center comes out clean. Cool on rack for 10 minutes. Use a knife to loosen bread; remove from pan. Serve warm or cool.

Store covered. Delicious sliced and toasted. Can be frozen up to 3 months.

Scones

Scones hail from Scotland and are a variation of a biscuit. With the addition of sugar, fruit and eggs (in the following recipes, egg whites or egg substitute), they are sweeter and more cakelike than biscuits. Scones are made basically the same way muffins and quick breads are mixed. Dry ingredients are combined. Wet ingredients are mixed, and then both mixtures are blended together. The batter should not be over mixed. Overmixing will make the scones tough.

The scone recipes in this cookbook have a minimum of fat and sugar. Butter and sugar are important ingredients that give scones their flavor and texture. Light butter (50% less fat than regular butter) and minimal amounts of sugar are used in the following recipes. You might want to use butter-flavored cooking spray to grease your baking pans.

Most of the scone recipes in this book contain fruit for natural sweetness. If the flavor is not sweet enough for you and additional sugar is no problem for your family's diet, increase the amount of sweetener used in the recipe.

Whole-wheat flour is included in each recipe for fiber, vitamins and nutrients. If you prefer not to use it, just use the same amount of all-purpose flour. I prefer using some whole-wheat flour in many of my recipes since it has more fiber than all-purpose flour.

Once the scone mixture holds together, gather dough into a ball, place on baking sheet which has been sprayed with cooking spray and pat into a circle, 8 or 9 inches, and about 1/2-inch thick. Using a sharp knife score the scone into wedges as per the directions in the recipe, being careful not to cut the dough all the way through. Bake according to directions.

Scones are done when they are golden brown and sound hollow when tapped. Remove the baked scones from the oven and cool about 5 minutes. When cool enough to handle, cut into wedges following the lines on the scone which you made before baking. Scones taste best served warm.

Store cooled scones in a covered container or a plastic bag at room temperature up to 3 days. Reheat in a 350°F oven for 5 to 10 minutes or until warmed. Or, toast in a toaster oven until warm. Baked scones can be frozen up to 3 months. Enjoy them as is or with a small amount of light butter or light margarine and/or jam of your choice.

BLUEBERRY CORNMEAL SCONES

CORNMEAL MAKES THESE SCONES FLAVORABLY FIBROUS
Prep time: 10 min   Baking time: 25 min
Makes: 1 Scone   Serving size: 1 Wedge, 1/12 Portion
Exchanges: 1 Starch and 1/2 Fat (1 Carbohydrate Choice)
Analysis per serving: 105 Calories, 20 g Carbohydrate, 3 g Protein,
2 g Fat, 4 mg Cholesterol, 160 mg Sodium, 2 g Fiber

3/4	cup whole-wheat flour
1/2	cup all-purpose flour
3/4	cup cornmeal
2	Tbs sugar
1	tsp baking powder
1/2	tsp baking soda
1/4	tsp salt
3	Tbs cold light butter or light magarine, cut into pieces
1	cup fresh or frozen blueberries, unthawed
1/2	tsp dried lemon peel or grated fresh lemon peel
2/3	cup buttermilk
1	tsp vanilla extract

Preheat oven 400°F. Spray baking sheet with cooking spray.

In medium bowl use a rubber spatula to combine flours, cornmeal, sugar, baking powder, baking soda, and salt. Cut in butter with pastry blender or two knives scissors-fashion until mixture resembles coarse crumbs. Use the spatula to stir in blueberries and lemon peel until berries are coated with flour mixture.

In 1-cup glass measuring cup, combine buttermilk and extract. With rubber spatula, stir into dry ingredients until batter is moistened and dough forms a ball.   Place dough ball on prepared baking sheet and pat into an 9-inch circle. Mark dough into 12 wedges, cutting into but not through dough. Bake 25 minutes or until golden brown. Cut into wedges and serve warm. Store covered and/or freeze up to 3 months.

To reheat, bake uncovered at 350°F for 5-10 minutes or toast in toaster oven until warm.

CHOCOLATE CHIP SCONES

THE ULTIMATE
Prep time: 10 min   Baking time: 20 min
Makes: 1 Scone   Serving size: 1 Wedge, 1/12 Portion
Exchanges: 1 Starch, 1/2 Fruit and 1/2 Fat (2 Carbohydrate Choices)
Analysis per serving: 136 Calories, 24 g Carbohydrate, 3 g Protein,
4 g Fat, 4 mg Cholesterol, 181 mg Sodium, 2 g Fiber

1	cup whole-wheat flour
1	cup all-purpose flour
2	tsp baking powder
1/2	tsp baking soda
1/4	tsp salt
1	Tbs sugar
1	Tbs brown sugar
3	Tbs cold light butter or light magarine
1/2	cup plain nonfat yogurt
1	tsp vanilla extract
1/3	cup mini chocolate chips

Preheat oven 400°F. Spray baking sheet with cooking spray.

In a medium bowl, combine flours, baking powder, salt and sugars. With pastry blender or two knives scissor-fashion, cut in butter until mixture resembles coarse crumbs. Using a rubber spatula, stir in yogurt, extract and chips until mixture holds together and forms a ball.

Place dough ball on prepared baking sheet. Pat into a 9-inch circle. Using a sharp knife, mark dough into 12 wedges, cutting into but not through dough.

Bake 20 minutes or until golden brown. Cut into wedges and serve warm. Or, cool and store covered and/or freeze up to 3 months.

To reheat, bake uncovered at 350°F for 5 to 10 minutes or toast in toaster oven until warm.

DELICIOUS DATE SCONES

DATES ADD NATURAL SWEETNESS, FLAVOR & TEXTURE
Prep time: 10 min   Bake time: 25 min
Makes: 1 Scone   Serving size: 1 Wedge, 1/12 Portion
Exchanges: 1 Starch, 1/2 Fruit and 1/2 Fat (2 Carbohydrate Choices)
Analysis per serving: 122 Calories, 24 g Carbohydrate, 4 g Protein,
2 g Fat, 4 mg Cholesterol, 267 mg Sodium, 3 g Fiber

1	cup whole-wheat flour
1	cup all-purpose flour
1/4	cup unprocessed wheat bran
2	Tbs brown sugar
2	tsp cinnamon
1 1/2	tsp baking powder
1 1/2	tsp baking soda
1/4	tsp salt
3	Tbs cold light butter or light magarine, cut into pieces
1/2	cup chopped dates
2/3	cup plain nonfat yogurt
1	tsp vanilla extract
2	large egg whites or 1/4 cup egg substitute

Preheat oven 350°F. Spray baking sheet with cooking spray.

In a medium bowl use a rubber spatula to combine flours, bran, brown sugar, cinnamon, baking powder, baking soda and salt; cut in butter with pastry blender or two knives scissor-fashion until mixture resembles coarse crumbs. Stir in dates until coated with flour mixture.

In a small bowl, use a whisk or a fork to combine yogurt, extract and egg whites. Add to dry ingredients, stirring with rubber spatula until blended and dough forms a ball.

Place ball of dough on prepared baking sheet. Sprinkle a little flour on dough and flatten into a 9-inch circle. Mark dough into 12 wedges, cutting into but not all the way through dough. Bake 25 to 28 minutes or until browned. Cut into wedges and serve warm. Or, cool and store covered and /or freeze up to 3 months.

To reheat, bake uncovered at 350°F 5 to 10 minutes or toast in toaster oven until warm.

GINGER SCONES

1	cup whole-wheat flour
1	cup all-purpose flour
2 1/2	tsp baking powder
1/2	tsp baking soda
1/4	tsp salt
3	Tbs sugar
3	tsp ginger
3	Tbs cold light butter or light magarine, cut into pieces
3/4	cup plain nonfat yogurt
1	tsp vanilla extract
2	large egg whites or 1/4 cup egg substitute
2	tsp dried orange peel or freshly grated orange peel

Preheat oven 400°F. Spray baking sheet with cooking spray.

In medium bowl, use a rubber spatula to combine flours, baking powder, baking soda, salt and ginger. Use a pastry blender or two knives scissor-fashion to cut in butter until mixture resembles coarse crumbs.

In small bowl, use a whisk or a fork to combine yogurt, egg whites and orange peel. Use a spatula to combine wet and dry ingredients until blended and dough forms a ball.

Put dough ball onto prepared baking sheet and pat into 9-inch circle. Use a sharp knife to mark dough into 12 wedges, cutting into but not through dough. Bake 20 minutes or until browned. Cut into wedges and serve warm. Or, store cooled wedges covered and/or freeze up to 3 months. To reheat, bake at 350°F for 5 to 10 minutes or toast in toaster oven until warm.

STRAWBERRY SCONES

SO GOOD
Prep time: 10 min   Baking time: 20 min
Makes: 1 Scone   Serving size: 1 Wedge, 1/12 Portion
Exchanges: 1 Starch and 1/2 Fat (1 Carbohydrate Choice)
Analysis per serving: 102 Calories, 19 g Carbohydrate, 3 g Protein,
2 g Fat, 4 mg Cholesterol, 136 mg Sodium, 2 g Fiber

1	**cup strawberries, washed, drained & hulled**
3	**Tbs sugar, divided**
1	**cup whole-wheat flour**
1	**cup all-purpose flour**
2	**tsp baking powder**
1/2	**tsp dried lemon peel or grated fresh lemon peel**
1/4	**tsp salt**
3	**Tbs cold light butter or light margarine**
1/2	**cup plain nonfat yogurt**

Cut strawberries into 1/2-inch pieces and toss with 1 Tbs sugar; set aside for 15 minutes.

Preheat oven 400°F. Spray baking sheet with cooking spray.

In a medium bowl, combine flours, baking powder, lemon peel, salt and remaining 2 Tbs sugar. With pastry blender or two knives scissor-fashion, cut in butter until mixture is crumbly. Add yogurt and strawberries with liquid and use a rubber spatula to combine ingredients until mixture holds together.

With floured hands, shape into a ball. Place ball on prepared baking sheet and pat into a 9-inch circle. Using a knife, mark dough into 12 wedges, cutting into but not through dough.

Bake about 20 minutes or until golden brown. Cut into wedges and serve warm. Or, store covered up to 2 days and/or freeze up to 3 months. To reheat, bake uncovered at 350°F for 5 to 10 or toast in toaster oven until warm.

Carbohydrate Counting and Exchange Lists

Careful meal planning is essential in managing blood glucose levels. Although there is no one diet for diabetes, nutritional recommendations changed drastically in 1994 when published studies gave priority to the toal amount of carbohydrate (CHO) rather than the source. Carbohydrate, the key nutrient in food that affects blood glucose levels, is the same whether it comes from bread, fruit or milk.

Scientific evidence shows that sucrose (table sugar) as part of a mealplan can be used by individuals with type I or type II diabetes without sacrificing blood glucose control. In fact, sucrose produces a glycemic response similiar to that of bread, rice and potatoes.*

Carbohydrate counting involves two steps; first identifying which foods contain carbohyrdate and next determining how many carbohydrate choices to count for each food. You may want to refer to the Exchange List chart on the next page. Use this equation to count the number of carbohydrate choices in a serving as:

1 carbohydrate choice = 15 grams of carbohydrate

Recipes in the DIABETIC GOODIE BOOK give serving sizes along with food exchanges and a complete nutrient profile to help determine how a serving of the recipe fits into your mealplan. Please note that if an ingredient is listed as (optional) in the recipe, its nutrient value is NOT calculated in the nutrient profile or Exchanges. If using the Exchange Lists for Mealplanning, use the following equation:

1 CHO choice = 15 g of CHO = 1 starch, fruit or milk exchange

The other two key nutrients, protein and fat do not affect blood glucose levels as much as carbohydrate, but are important for good nutrition and calorie control. It is important to follow your mealplan as determined by your physician and registered dietitian, eating about the same amount of protein each day.

Fat, on the other hand, is generally controlled for good cardiovascular health and can be incorporated into carbohydrate counting by using these guidelines.

One carbohydrate choice (7-22 g CHO) can have 3 g or less fat. Two carbohydrate choices (23-37 g CHO) can have 6 g or less fat. Three carbohydrate choices (38-52 g CHO) can have 9 g or less fat, and four carbohydrate choices (53-65 g CHO) can have up to 12 g of fat.

The American Dietetic Association and the American Diabetes Association have grouped foods together with like amounts of carbohydrates, protein and fat. The following chart shows the amount of nutrients in one serving from each list.

Groups/Lists	CHO (g)	Protein (g)	Fat (g)	Calories
Carbohydrate Group				
Starch	15	3	1 or less	80
Fruit	15	---	---	60
Milk				
Skim	12	8	0-3	90
Low-fat	12	8	5	120
Whole	12	8	8	150
Other CHOs	15	varies	varies	varies
Vegetables	5	2	---	25
Meat and Meat Substitute Group				
Very Lean	---	7	0-1	35
Lean	---	7	3	55
Medium-fat	---	7	5	75
High-fat	---	7	8	100
Fat Group	---	---	5	45

For more information regarding Meal Planning, Exchange List Food Groups, Carbohydrate Counting and Nutritional Recommendations for Diabetes Management, please call or write the following organizations:

American Dietetic Association
216 W. Jackson Blvd.
Chicago, IL 60606
#800/366-1655

American Diabetes Association
1660 Duke Street
Alexandria, VA 22314
#800/232-3472

*JOURNAL OF THE AMERICAN DIETETIC ASSOCIATION. "Nutrition Recommendations and Principles for People with Diabetes Mellitus." 1994. 94(5):504-506.

The New Food Label at a Glance

The new food label will carry an up-to-date, easier-to-use nutrition information guide, to be required on almost all packaged foods (compared to about 60 percent of products up till now). The guide will serve as a key to help in planning a healthy diet.*

Serving sizes are now more consistent across product lines, stated in both household and metric measures, and reflect the amounts people actually eat.

The **list of nutrients** covers those most important to the health of today's consumers, most of whom need to worry about getting too much of certain items (fat, for example), rather than too few vitamins or minerals, as in the past.

The label of larger packages must now tell the number of calories per gram of fat, carbohydrate, and protein.

Nutrition Facts

Serving Size ½ cup (114g)

Servings Per Container 4

Amount Per Serving

Calories 90	Calories from Fat 30

	% Daily Value*
Total Fat 3g	**5%**
Saturated Fat 0g	**0%**
Cholesterol 0mg	**0%**
Sodium 300mg	**13%**
Total Carbohydrate 13g	**4%**
Dietary Fiber 3g	**12%**
Sugars 3g	
Protein 3g	

Vitamin A	80%	•	Vitamin C	60%
Calcium	4%	•	Iron	4%

* Percent Daily Values are based on a 2,000 calorie diet. Your daily values may be higher or lower depending on your calorie needs:

		Calories	2,000	2,500
Total Fat	Less than		65g	80g
Sat Fat	Less than		20g	25g
Cholesterol	Less than		300mg	300mg
Sodium	Less than		2,400mg	2,400mg
Total Carbohydrate			300g	375g
Fiber			25g	30g

Calories per gram:

Fat 9 • Carbohydrate 4 • Protein 4

New title signals that the label contains the newly required information.

Calories from fat are now shown on the label to help consumers meet dietary guidelines that recommend people get no more than 30 percent of their calories from fat.

% Daily Value shows how a food fits into the overall daily diet.

Daily Values are also something new. Some are maximums, as with fat (65 grams or less); others are minimums, as with carbohydrate (300 grams or more). The daily values for a 2,000- and 2,500-calorie diet must be listed on the label of larger packages. Individuals should adjust the values to fit their own calorie intake.

* This label is only a sample. Exact specifications are in the final rules.
Source: Food and Drug Administration 1993

Nutrition Claims

Manufacturers use eye-catching claims such as light or lite, free, low, reduced, less and high to give their products a competitive edge. Here are key nutrition terms and their meanings as defined by the government.

Calorie-free: less than 5 calories per serving.

Low-calorie: 40 calories or less per serving.

Reduced-calorie/fewer calories: distinguishes foods having calories per serving reduced by 25% or more.

Light/lite/lightly: has at least one-third fewer calories or 50% less fat than its counterparts. When describi ng color, texture or taste, the particular characteristic MUST be identified. For example, an olive oil bottle must read that it is "light" in color since no oil as of yet is truly "light" in calories or fat.

Fat-free/no-fat/nonfat: no more that 0.5 gram of fat per serving.

Low-fat: 3 grams of fat or less per serving.

Lowfat: refers to milk or milk products that have "some" milk fat removed. Milk percentages, such a 1% and 2%, describe the fat volume not the fat calories. (Note that lowfat is one word when describing milk. It becomes two words when associated with other foods.) Inspect milk labels carefully for fat content as they are highly variable. For instance, 2% lowfat milk has 5 grams of fat per cup, while 1/2 percent drops to .5 gram.

Reduced-fat/less fat: at least 25% less fat that its original counterpart.

Saturated fat-free: less than .5 gram of saturated fat per serving and the level of trans fatty acids does not exceed 1% of total fat.

Low in saturated fat: the cutoff point for this descriptor is 1 gram saturated fat per serving and not more than 15% of calories from saturated fat.

Reduced/less saturated fat: at least 25% less saturated fat than its original counterpart with a minimum reduction of 1 gram saturated fat per serving.

Cholesterol-free/no cholesterol: less than 2 milligrams of cholesterol AND 2 grams or less of saturated fat per serving. Other analogous terms are "no cholesterol" and "zero cholesterol."

Low-cholesterol/low in cholesterol: no more than 20 milligrams of cholesterol and 2 grams or less of saturated fat per serving.

Reduced-cholesterol/less cholesterol: cholesterol is cut by 25% or more. The reduction must be at least 20 milligrams per servings.

Lean/extra lean: for meat, poultry, seafood and game meat. "Lean" describes products with no more than 10 grams of fat, 4 grams of saturated fat and 95 milligrams of cholesterol per 100 grams cooked weight (about 3 1/2 ounces). "Extra lean" meat contains less than 5 grams of fat, less than 2 grams of saturated fat and less than 95 milligrams of cholesterol per 100 grams cooked weight.

Sugar-free: less than .5 gram of total sugar per serving.

Reduced-sugar/less sugar: at least 25% less sugar than its original counterpart.

Sodium-free/salt-free: no more than 5 milligrams of sodium per serving and does not contain sodium chloride (table salt).

Very low/low-sodium: 35 milligrams of sodium or less per serving. "Low" describes 140 milligrams of sodium or less per serving.

Reduced-sodium/less sodium: at least 25% less sodium than its original counterpart.

Light/lite in sodium: 50% less sodium than its original counterpart.

More/fortified/enriched/added: describe a food that contains at least 10% more of the Daily Value for protein, fiber, vitamins or minerals than does a comparable equivalent.

Contact the following agencies for more information on nutrition labels or for answers regarding food and nutrition:

American Dietetic Association Consumer Nutrition Hotline #800-366-1655

FDA/USDA Food Labeling Education Information Center #301-504-5719 Fax #301-504-6409

Healthy Hints For Snacking

Set a good example for the entire family. Teach the family good nutritional habits.

Limit the amount of junk food in the house. Serve homemade snacks because you can control what goes into the snacks if you prepare them yourself.

Don't use food as a pacifier, reward or punishment. Food should not have an emotional value.

Set limits, but make them reasonable. Be willing to compromise. Forbidding a food only makes it more enticing.

Teach yourself and your family to enjoy food in moderation. Don't label food "good" or "bad."

Cut back on purchasing sweet and salty snacks. Most are laden with fat and come with unwanted, excess calories.

Read all package labels. Check for hidden salt, sugar and fat. Remember: the term "natural" does not mean salt- or sugar-free. The caloric value may even be higher. Ingredients are listed by their prominence by weight on the label.

Don't deny a sweet tooth. Experiment with fruit to sweeten. You not only get a sweet taste, but you get fiber as a bonus.

Decrease your family's intake of caffeine and sugar which can trigger the release of insulin, causing blood sugar levels to drop and produce feelings of hunger. Use unsweetened, flavored waters and seltzers. Try to drink at least 8 glasses of water a day. A lemon slice added to a glass of cold water is very refreshing.

Brush your teeth immediately after each meal. It will help you keep from snacking.

Reasons for Imperfect Cookies

Cookies irregular in size and shape: Improperly dropped or overbaked

Edges dark and crusty: Cookie sheet too large for oven

Dry, hard cookies: Overbaked cookies

Doughy cookies: Underbaked cookies

Excessive spreading: Dough too warm. Baking sheet too hot. Oven temperature incorrect. Undermeasurement of dry ingredients.

What Happened To My Cake?

	Shortening Cake	Sponge-Type Cake
Coarse grain	-Used all-purpose flour instead of cake flour -Excess leavening -Not enough creaming -Undermixing -Baking temperature too low	-Used all-purpose flour instead of cake flour -Excess leavening -Not enough creaming -Undermixing
Heaviness/ Too Compact	-Excess of liquid, shortening or eggs -Not enough flour or leavening -Overmixing -Baking temperature too high	-Underbeaten egg yolks or overbeaten egg whites -Overmixing
Heavy, soggy layer at bottom	-Excess liquid -Shortening too soft -Underbeaten eggs -Undermixing -Baking time too short	-Excess of eggs or egg yolks -Underbeaten egg yolks -Failure to bake batter properly after turning into pan -Underbeating
Hard top crust	-Baking temperature too high -Baking time too long	-Baking temperature too high -Baking time too long
Cracked or humped top	-Excess flour -Not enough liquid -Overmixing -Uneven spreading of batter -Baking temperature too high	-Excess flour or sugar -Baking temperature too high

	Shortening Cake	Sponge-Type Cake
Sticky top crust	-Excess sugar -Baking time too short	-Excess sugar -Baking time too short
Falling	-Excess sugar, liquid, leavening or shortening	-Excess sugar -Overbeaten egg whites -Incomplete mixing
Tough crumb	-Not enough sugar -Not enough shortening -Excess flour -Excess eggs -Baking temperature too high -Overmixing	-Not enough sugar -Underbeaten egg yolk or egg whites -Omission of cream of tartar (Angel Food Cake) -Excess eggs -Baking temperature too high -Baking time too long
Crumbling or falling apart	-Excess sugar, leavening or shortening -Undermixing -Incorrect preparation of pan -Incorrect cooling	
Falling out of pan before cooling is complete		-Baking time too short -Excess sugar -Greasing of pan
One side higher	-Uneven spreading of batter -Pan warped -Range or oven rack not level -Pan too close to wall of oven -Uneven oven heat	-Pan warped -Range or oven rack not level
Pale top crust	-Baking temperature too low -Not enough sugar or shortening -Excess flour -Pan too large -Overmixing	-Baking temperature too low -Overbeaten egg whites -Baking time too long

Some cakes may not be successful because of failure to beat and add egg whites and egg yolks separately where a recipe directs. Follow directions of each recipe precisely and carefully. Adding whole eggs, no matter how thoroughly beaten, may produce different results.

Freezer Hints and Storage Times

Do not freeze custard or cream pies.

Unbaked pies: prepare fruit pies according to directions. Do not cut vents in top crust until ready to bake. Wrap, label, and freeze. To bake: unwrap pie; make slits in top crust, place unthawed in preheated oven (at temperature specified in recipe) and bake allowing 10 to 15 minutes longer than recipe time.

Baked pies: prepare according to recipe. Cool completely. Wrap, label, and freeze. Thaw and warm at 375°F for 30 to 40 minutes.

Chiffon pies: prepare according to recipe. Wrap, label, and freeze. Defrost in refrigerator.

Unbaked cobblers or tarts: prepare according to directions. Wrap, label, and freeze. Place unthawed in preheated oven (at temperature specified in recipe) and bake allowing 10 to 15 minutes longer than recipe time.

Baked cobblers or tarts: prepare according to recipe. Cool completely. Wrap, label, and freeze. Thaw and warm at 375°F for 30 to 40 minutes.

Cookies: Bake and cool according to recipe. Place waxed paper between layers. Freeze airtight and label. Defrost at room temperature. Refrigerated dough cookies: form unbaked dough into rolls and wrap securely in freezer wrap; label. Defrost in refrigerator and bake according to recipe.

Cheesecake: Prepare according to recipe and bake. Cool completely. Wrap securely, label and freeze. Place in refrigerator to thaw. Do not thaw at room temperature.

Cake: Prepare according to recipe and bake. Cool completely. Wrap securely, label and freeze. Thaw at room temperature.

Coffee Cake: Wrap cooled cake securely or seal in freezer bag; label and freeze. Thaw at room temperature or place on paper plate and defrost in microwave about 10 minutes, rotating every 3 minutes until defrosted and/or warm. Can be reheated in preheated 350°F oven for 5 to 10 minutes. Best served warm.

Muffins: Wrap cooled muffins securely or seal in freezer bag; label. Thaw at room temperature or place on paper plate and defrost in microwave about 5 to 10 minutes depending upon amount of muffins defrosted. Rotate every 3 minutes until defrosted and/or warm. If desired, split and toast.

Quick Bread: Wrap cooled bread securely or seal in freezer bag; label. Thaw at room temperature or place on paper plate and defrost in microwave about 10 minutes, rotating every 3 minutes until defrosted and/or wa rm. Can be reheated in preheated 350°F oven for 5 to 10 minutes. Or, defrost and slice and toast.

Scones: Wrap cooled scones securely or seal in freezer bag; label. Defrost at room temperature or place on paper plate and defrost in microwave 5 to 10 minutes, rotating every 3 minutes until defrosted and/or warm. Or, defrost, reheat in 350°F oven 5 to 10 minutes or toast in toaster oven. Serve warm.

Please note that when preparing food for freezer storage, be sure that all air is removed from wrap, container or freezer bag so that when it is defrosted it will retain the original fresh flavor and texture. To prevent freezer burn, all items placed in freezer must be securely wrapped or sealed without air pockets.

Pies:	unbaked	6 months
	baked	6 months
	chiffon	2 months
Coffee Cakes:	baked	3 months
Cobblers & Tarts:	unbaked	6 months
	baked	6 months
Cakes:	butter-type	4 months
	angel food	6 to 8 months
	sponge	6 to 8 months
	with fruit	6 months
Cheesecakes:	baked	3 months
Cookies & Bars:	baked	12 months
Muffins:	baked	3 months
Quick Breads:	baked	3 months
Scones:	baked	3 months

Fruit Chart

Apples
All year, Aug to Nov.
Peak: Oct
All purpose: Granny-Smith, Mackintosh, Cortland, Golden Delicious
Cooking: Rome Beauty
Eating: Red Delicious
Firm, heavy, well-colored
Minor patches or brownish skin does not affect quality
Refrigerate

Apricots
Late May - early April
Plump, fairly firm. Deep yellow or yellow-orange.
Yields gently to pressure.
Deep aroma.
Very firm & greenish fruit will not ripen.
Use overripe fruit immediately
Refrigerate

Bananas
All year Peak: Dec - May
Firm to slightly soft, heavy for size.
Irregular brown marks do not affect quality.
Best not to refrigerate.
Refrigerate 1 or 2 days to prevent overripening.
The riper the fruit the sweeter it is.
Brush cut surfaces w/ lemon juice to prevent discoloring.
High sugar content.

Berries
Blackberries, boysenberries, loganberries & raspberries
June - Aug
Peak: July
Plump, fresh appearing, uniform & well-colored.
Avoid moldy spots.
Refrigerate well-ventilated in basket or spread out on trays.
Very perishable, use ASAP.
Can be frozen in air-tight container.
Frozen berries need not be thawed before use in recipes.

Blueberries
Late May to late Sept
Peak: July
Plump, clear colors
Avoid moldy ones
Refrigerate as other berries.
Keep in fridge up to 1 week.
High sugar content.

Cherries
Sweet & Sour May - Aug
Peak: June - July
Plump, firm from bright red to black.
Reject cherries w/blemishes or brown spots.
Refrigerate w/stems.
Perishable.
Wash and drain before destemming.
Darker color indicates sweeter fruit.
High sugar content.

Dates
All year
Fresh dates are soft, plump and smooth.
Cover and refrigerate.
Fresh & dried can be used interchangeably.
High sugar content.

Figs
Early June - early Nov
Soft, greenish yellow, purple or black.
Refrigerate, extremely perishable.
Freeze in airtight container.
High sugar content.

Grapefruit
All year, primarily Oct - June
Firm & springy to touch, heavy for size.
Color varies.
Quality is not affected if tinged w/green.
Store at room temperature for a few days or refrigerate for longer storage.

Grapes
All year
Peak: Sept
Popular varieties: Concord, Ribier,
Thompson seedless, Tokay Smooth,
plump.
Firmly attached to stem.
Refrigerate in perforated plastic bag.
Wash, drain & freeze on sheets.
Store in plastic bag.
Eat frozen.
High sugar content.

Kiwi
All year
Fuzzy, leathery skin.
Firm but yields to pressure.
Should be soft.
Reject wrinkled fruit.
Refrigerate in plastic bag.
Tart, sweet flavor.
Peel skin and slice.

Mangos
May - Aug
Firm to soft.
Yields to pressure.
Heady aroma.
Reject wrinkled ones.
May be green, yellow or tinged with red.
Refrigerate.
Peel, slice & cube.
High sugar content.

Melons
Cantaloupe
May - Sept
Rounded with rough veined scars.
Sweet aroma when ripe.
Refrigerate

Casaba
July - Nov
Peak: Sept - Oct
Yellow rind.
Slight softening at end.
Sweet cucumber-like aroma.
Refrigerate.

Cranshaw
July - Oct
Peak: Aug - Sept
Golden rind.
Slight softening near stem.

Rich, slightly spicy aroma.
Refrigerate.

Honeydew
Primarily Jun - Oct
Creamy color, velvety rind.
May have slight softening at stem end.
Delicate fruity aroma.
Refrigerate.

Watermelon
May - Sept
Peak: July - Aug
Flesh should be bright & firm.
Hard seeds.
Refrigerate.
High sugar content.

Nectarines
Mid May - late Sept
Peak: July - Aug
Plump, bright, firm but not hard.
Golden color.
Delicate aroma.
Avoid hard, dull or very soft fruit.
Refrigerate.

Oranges
Temple: Oct - Dec
Valencia: Mar - July
Firm, heavy for size.
Avoid puffy or spongy fruit.
Store a few days at room temperature or
refrigerate several weeks.
Navel: popular eating - no seeds.
Valencia: juice orange.
High sugar content.

Peaches
Mid May - late Sept
Peak: July - Aug
Bright, firm, creamy to golden color.
Strong fragrance.
Yields to pressure.
Reject fruit with green color - will not ripen
well.
Refrigerate.

Pears

Bartlett: July - Nov
Anjou, Bosc, Comece: Sept - Mar
Seckel: Sept - Dec
Firm.
Yields to pressure.
Refrigerate when fruit yields to pressure.
Great w/cheese.

Pineapple

All year
Peak: Mar - June
Plump, heavy for size.
Sweet fragrance when ripe.
Firm, fresh appearance.
Softening is sign of deterioration.
Use ASAP.
Best not to refrigerate until just before serving.
Refrigerate to prevent overripening.
Freeze in airtight container.

Plums

Italian prune, Santa Rosa, Weckson
Late May - mid Sept
Fairly firm to slightly soft.
Yields to gentle pressure.
Reject hard, poorly colored or shriveled fruit.
Ripen quickly.
Use overripe fruit ASAP.
Refrigerate.
Freeze in airtight container.

Strawberries

All year
Peak: April - June
Plump, natural shine, rich red with green caps.
Refrigerate with caps in ventilated basket or spread on trays.
Use ASAP.
Freeze in airtight container.
Wash with caps on just before using; then drain & hull.

Glossary

BAKE - Cook in oven until cooked and browned, i.e. cookies, cakes, etc.

BEAT - Make mixture smooth by vigorous over and over motion with spoon, fork, whisk, rotary beater or electric mixer

BLEND - Thoroughly combine all ingredients until very smooth and uniform

BRUSH - Spread food with a liquid ingredient using a small brush

BUBBLY - When food has come to a boil and bubbles

BUTTERMILK BAKING MIX - Packaged baking mix such as Low-Fat Bisquick Baking Mix or Insta-Bake Whole-Wheat Baking Mix by Hodgson Mill. Insta-Bake is lower in fat, sodium and carbohydrate than Bisquick. Both buttermilk baking mixes can be purchased in most food stores in the aisle with flour and sugar.

CHILL - Cool in refrigerator

CHOP - Cut into small pieces

COAT - Roll in flour, nuts, sugar, crumbs, etc. until all surfaces are covered

COBBLER - Deep-dish fruit pie with top crust only

COMBINE - Mix all ingredients together

COOK - Prepare food by applying heat in any form

COOL - Allow all heated items come to room temperature

CREAM - Beat until soft and smooth usually with electric mixer

CRUMBLY - Combine all ingredients so that mixture looks like small peas

CUT IN - Mix fat (butter, margarine, oil) into flour mixture with pastry blender, fork or two knives

DASH - A small amount

DEFROST - Leave frozen food at room temperature or in refrigerator until it is no longer frozen

DOT - Scatter small amounts of butter, nuts, etc. over surface of food

DRAIN - Pour off all liquid, usually through a strainer, while reserving food product

DUST - Sprinkle a food lightly with sugar or flour

FOLD - Mix gently by lifting batter or mixture from bottom to top with a rubber spatula

FIRM - Having a solid texture

FROTHY - Bubbly

GRADUALLY - A little at a time

GREASE - Spray bottom and sides of cooking or baking utensil with cooking spray to prevent food product from sticking

HULL - Pluck out green stem and leaves of strawberry

INGREDIENT - A food item used in recipe

LEAVENING - Baking powder or baking soda used in baked goods to produce a gas that lightens batter

LIGHT - Not thick or heavy

LINE - Cover inside of pan with waxed paper, parchment paper or aluminum foil. Line muffin tins with pap er liners

LUKEWARM - Cool enough to touch

MARINATE - Let food stand in liquid to add flavor

MASH - Flatten with fork until soft and smooth

MELT - Heat until product turns to liquid

MERINGUE - Egg whites beaten stiff with sugar and baked

MIX - Stir ingredients together

PARE - Cut off outer covering with knife or peeler, i.e. apples, pears, carrots, etc.

PEAKS - Soft or stiff. Mixture that stands up when beaters are lifted from contents of bowl

PEEL - Strip off outer covering, i.e. banana, orange, avocado, etc.

PHYLLO - A tissue-thin leaf of sheets of dough, usually layered when used in food preparation

PRECOOKED - Already cooked

PROCESS - Turn on food processor or blender and combine ingredients

PULSE - Turn food processor on and off with short, quick motions

QUARTER - Cut food into four equal parts

REFRIGERATE - Store or chill in refrigerator

ROLL OUT - Flatten and spread with rolling pin

SCORE - Cut top layer with knife in a crisscross pattern

SCRAPE - Use a rubber spatula to remove batter or mixture from sides of bowl, incorporating into contents of bowl

SEPARATE - Divide into parts

SERRATED KNIFE - Knife with ridges in blade

SERVING - Quantity of food needed for one person

SET - Firm, no longer loose and liquid, especially in recipes using gelatin

SHRED - Cut into thin pieces using a grater, shredder or food processor

SIFT - Put dry ingredients through a sifter or fine sieve

SKIN - Peel outer layer of skin from fruit

SLICE - Cut in thin, flat pieces with a knife

SMOOTH - When mixture is free of lumps and ingredients are incorporated

SOFTEN - Leave food at room temperature so it becomes soft

SOFTLY BEATEN EGG WHITES - Egg whites (or pasteurized dry egg whites) which have been at room temperature for at least 30 minutes and beaten at high speed with an electric mixer. Softly beaten egg whites will hold their shape softly but will droop when beaters are lifted or when lifted with a rubber spatula. If you tilt the bowl, the egg whites will slide around.

SPLIT - Divide evenly into two pieces or parts

SPREAD - Cover surface smoothly with a thin layer of ingredients

SPRINKLE - Scatter one ingredient on top of another

STIFF - Batter sticks up straight and holds its shape when beaters are lifted

STIFFLY BEATEN EGG WHITES - Egg whites (or pasteurized dry egg whites) which have been at room temperature for at least 30 minutes and beaten at high speed with an electric mixer. Egg whites are stiffly beaten when they are glossy and dense and hold their shape when beaters are lifted or when whites are lifted with a rubber spatula. They will remain firm and not droop. Stiffly beaten egg whites will not move if you tilt the bowl. If you overbeat stiffly beaten egg whites, they will become lumpy and grainy and you must start all over again with new ingredients.

STIR - Combine ingredients with a circular motion until uniform consistency

SWIRL - Drop mounds of a second mixture on top of first mixture and use a knife to marbleize by cutting through both mixtures

SUBSTITUTE - Use one food or ingredient in place of another

TEASPOONFUL - Use a measuring teaspoon to measure ingredients; use a tableware teaspoon to drop batter onto baking sheet

THICKEN - Make liquid mixture become more dense

TOP - Place an ingredient above another

TOSS - Tumble ingredients lightly with a lifting motion

UTENSIL - Kitchen tool used in cooking and baking

WELL - When dry ingredients have been pushed to sides of bowl and a hollow is formed in middle of ingredients

WHIRL - Combine ingredients in food processor

WHIP - Beat with electric mixer to add air and volume

YOGURT CHEESE - Drained yogurt that has thickened and looks like cream cheese; see also page 9 or 83

INDEX

Diabetic Goodie Book

Diabetic Goodie Book

DIABETIC GOODIE BOOK by Kathy Kochan. Over 190 recipes for desserts and baked goodies. Each formulated with an awareness of fat, sugar, salt, cholesterol, carbohydrate and protein with exchanges and nutrient analyses. Plus, kitchen tips, substitutions, nutrition claims and other helpful information. 256 pages, Softcover. $15.95 each.........Send me____at $_____

COOKING ALA HEART More than 90,000 copies in print, its recipes are always hailed as original, delicious and easy to make. Selected by the editors of the Harvard Medical School health letter. Two chapters of sound nutrition information and over 400 recipes! 456 pages, Softcover. $19.95 each.........Send me____at $_____

HEALTHY MEXICAN COOKING 140 authentic low-fat recipes for delicious, traditional Mexican foods. Few ingredients, practical preparations and moderate to low calories. Glossary and special mail-order section. Diabetic exchanges and full nutrient analyses. 256 pages, Softcover. $14.95 each........Send me____at $_____

THE ESSENTIAL ARTHRITIS COOKBOOK Ktichen Basics for people with arthritis, fibromyalgia and other chronic pain and fatigue. Excellent nutrition information, medication tables, photos and more. 120 low-fat recipes that save time and energy! 288 pages, Hardcover. $24.95 each........Send me____at $_____

WHAT'S FOR BREAKFAST? The easiest way to stop cheating yourself out of a good breakfast. Over 100 recipes, easy and delicious. Super Quick, Quick and Worth the Effort. Sound nutrition and Pro-Carb Connection! 288 pages, Softcover. $13.95 each.........Send me____at $_____

GIFTS OF THE HEART Reprinted and revised. Delightful recipes and gift ideas from Fudge Sauce to Barbecue Sauce, Cookies and Snacks, even Soups and Breads. Cute addition to a gift basket, perfect as a thank you or forget-me-not. 64 pages, Softcover. $8.50 each...........Send me____at $_____

SHIPPING
Add $4.00 for one book, $5.00/2 books, $6.00/3 books, $7.00/4-6 books...........................$_____

Minnesota residents must add sales tax...6.5% tax $_____

TOTAL ENCLOSED $_____

Circle Method of Payment: Check   Visa   Master Card

Card Number _____Exp Date_____

Name_____

PO Box and/or Street Address_____

_____

City, State and Zip Code_____

Mail to: APPLETREE PRESS INC. 151 GOOD COUNSEL DRIVE MANKATO, MN 56001
Call Toll Free #800-322-5679 or Fax Your Order to #507-345-3002 Local calls #507-345-4848